Drug Metabolism

Edited by Katherine Dunnington

Published in London, United Kingdom

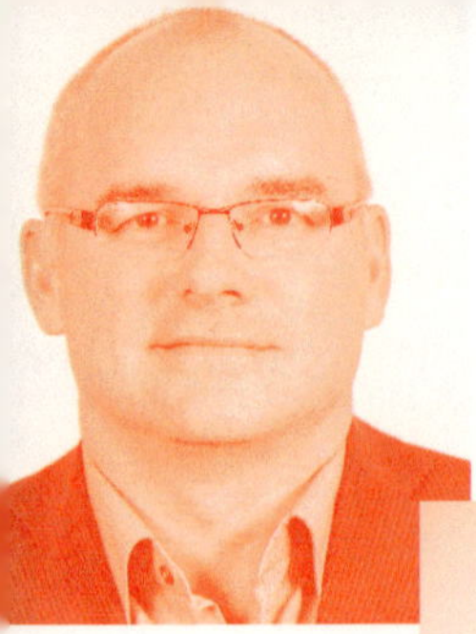
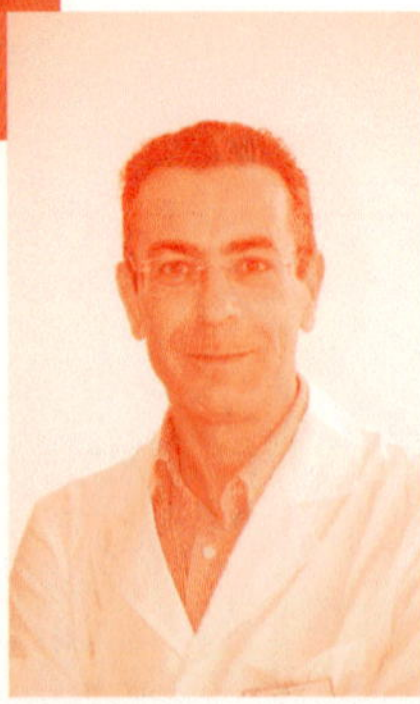
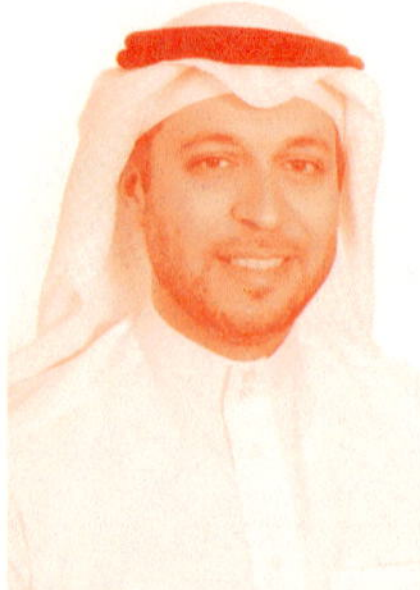
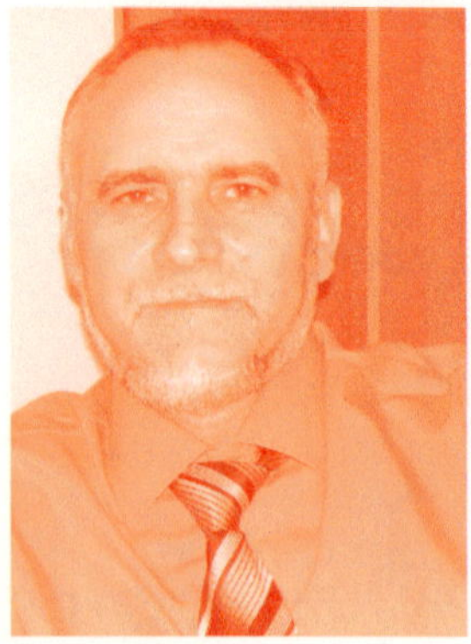
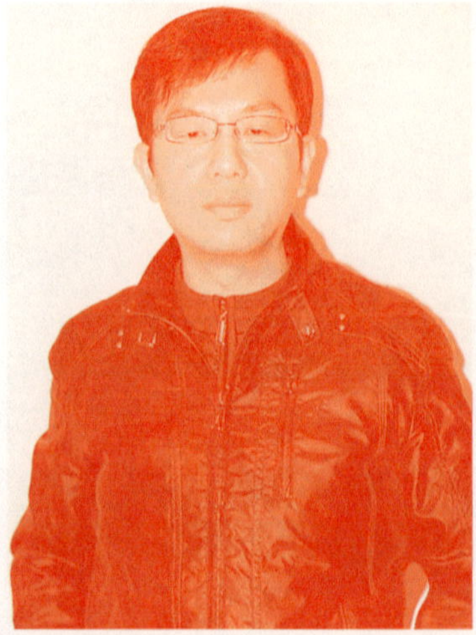
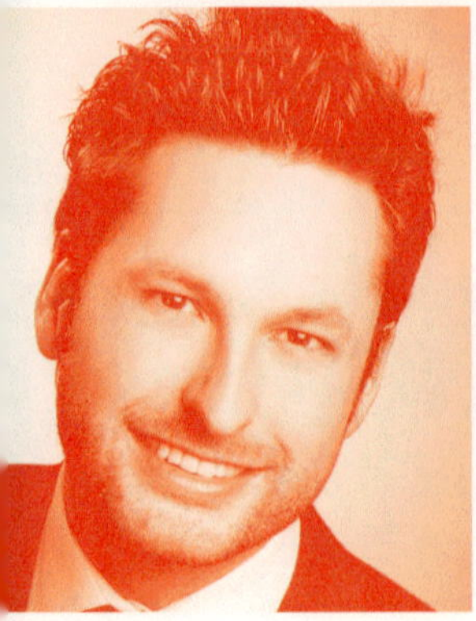
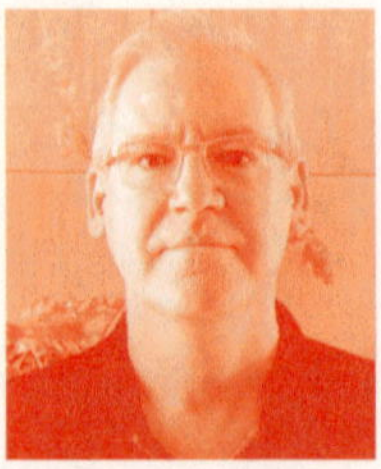

IntechOpen

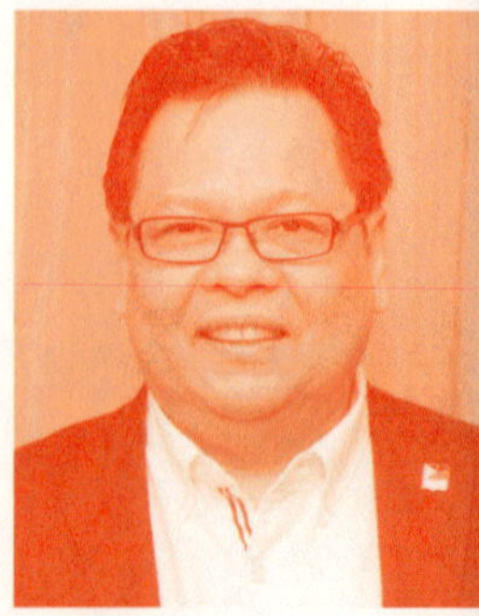
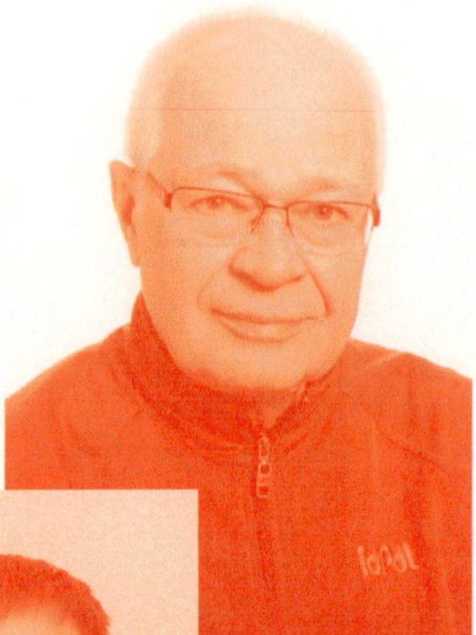
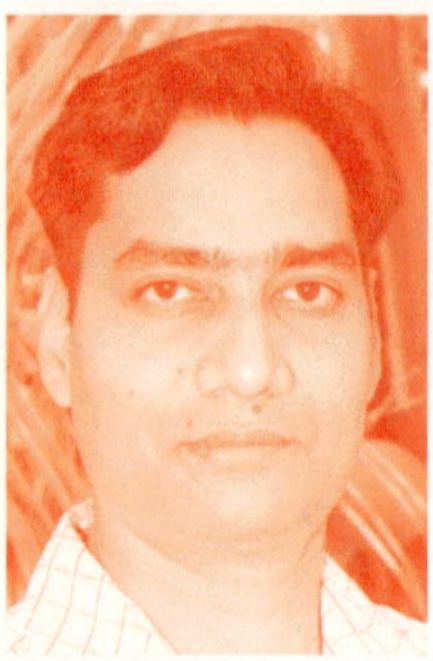
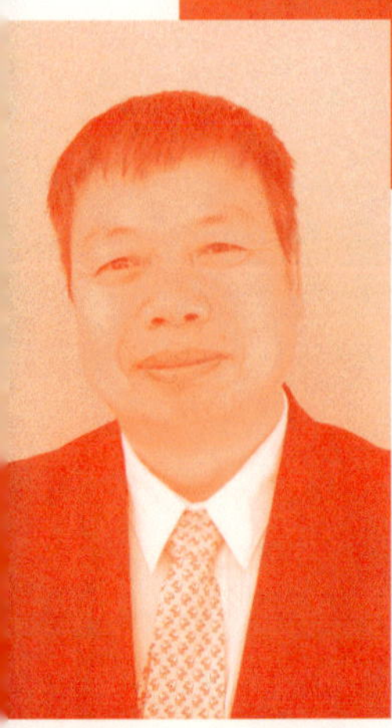
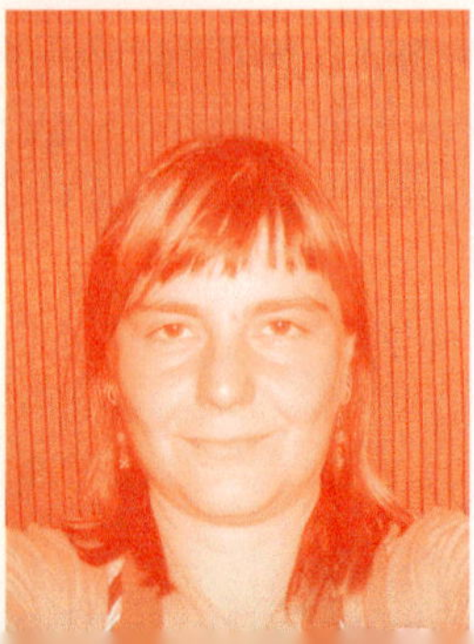
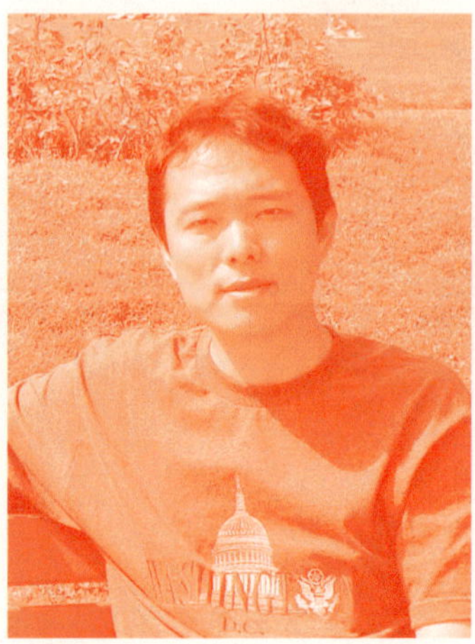

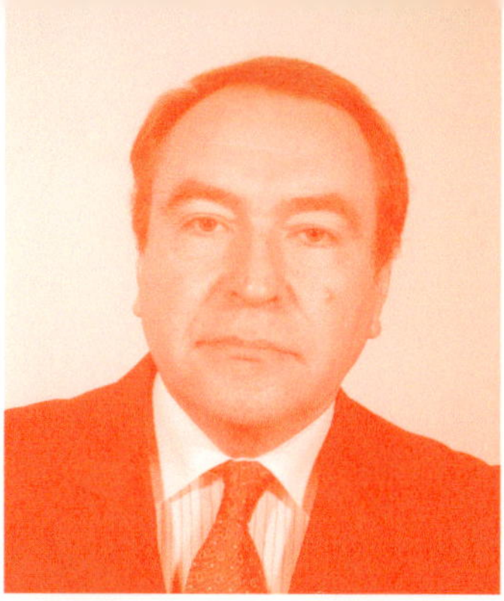
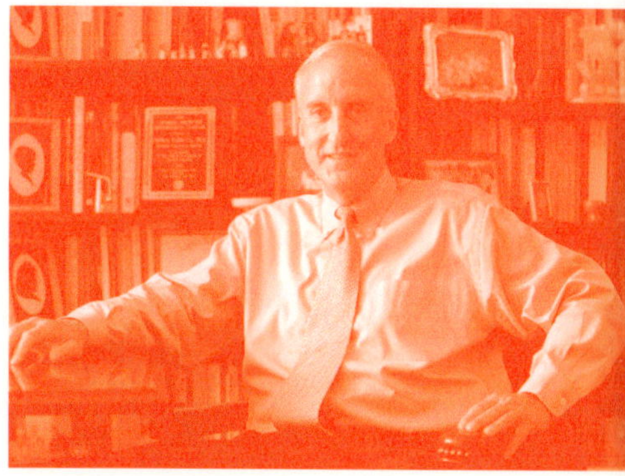
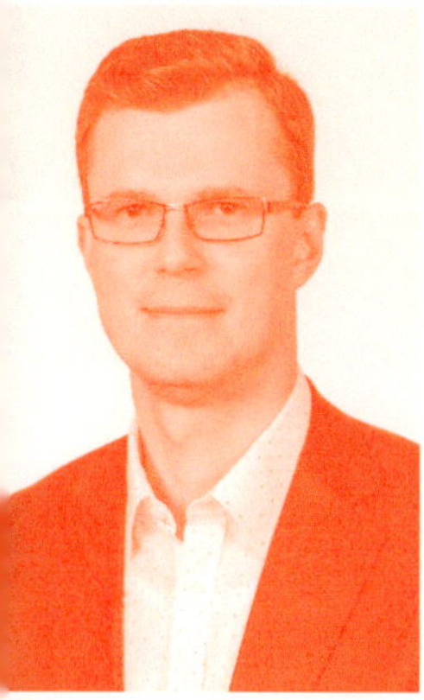
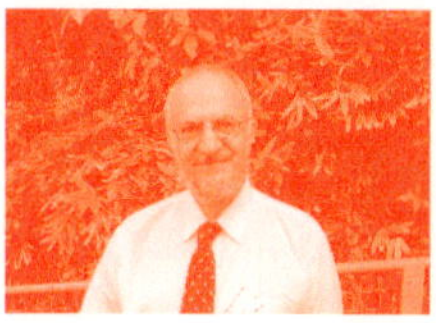
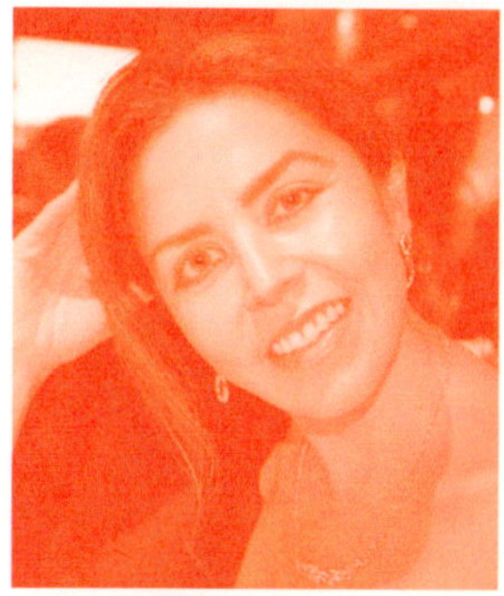

Supporting open minds since 2005

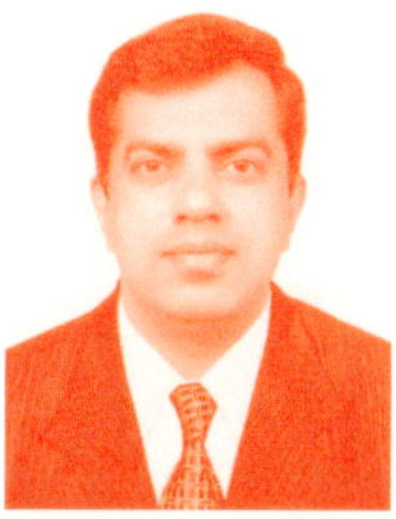
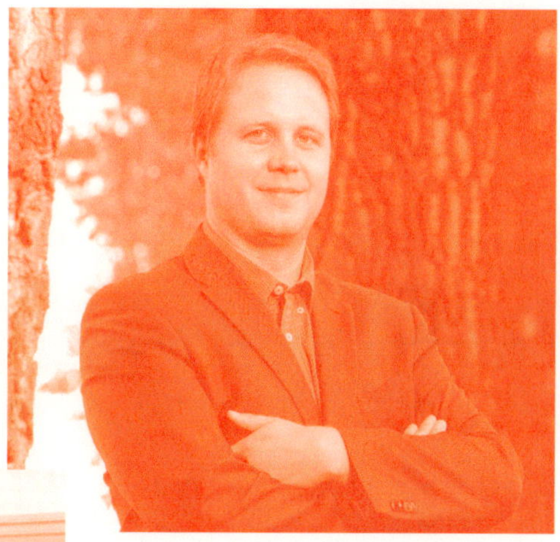
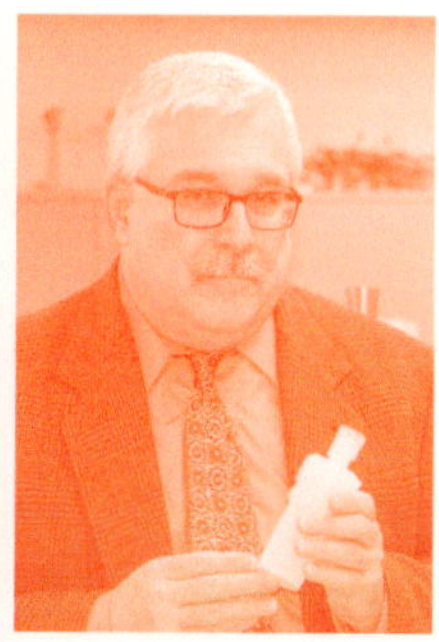
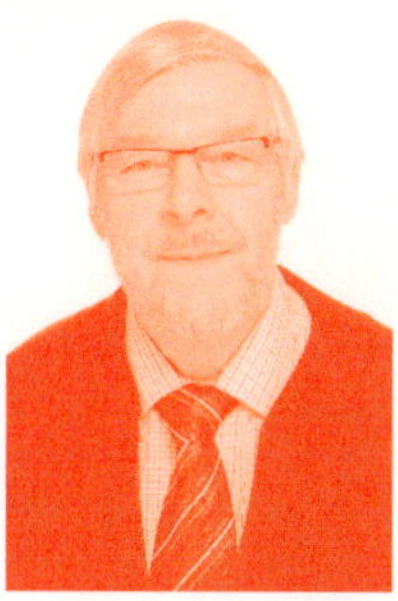
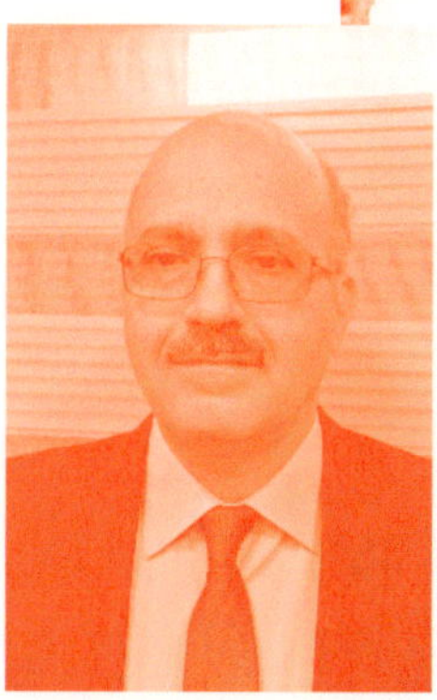
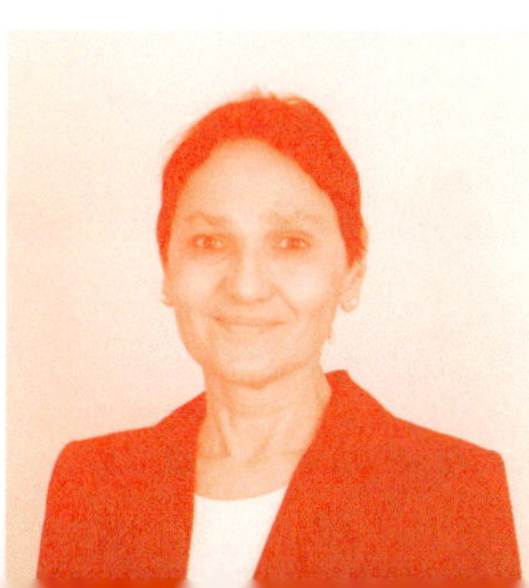
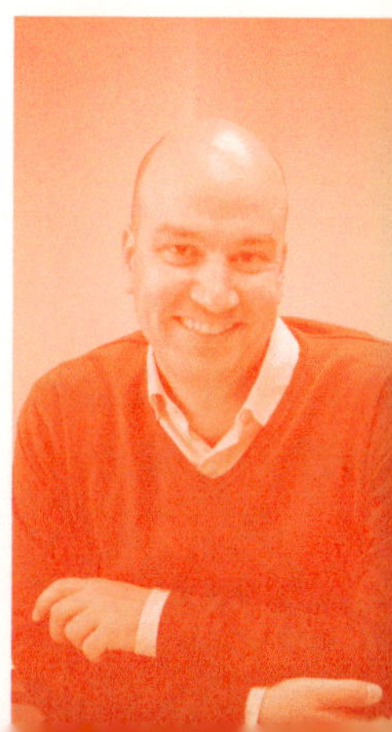

Drug Metabolism
http://dx.doi.org/10.5772/intechopen.91543
Edited by Katherine Dunnington

Contributors
Guadalupe Ortiz-Lopez, Katy Sanchez-Pozos, Maria De Los Angeles Granados-Silvestre, Selvan Ravindran, Tanu Dixit, Akash Tiwari, Sneha Bose, Himani Kulkarni, Jitendra Suthar, Vamsi Krishna Marothu, Kantamaneni Padmalatha, Gorrepati Madhavi, Benjamin Mann, Roger Melton, David Thompson, Shweta Dutta, Sarawati Prasad Mishra, Anil Kumar Kumar Sahu, Koushlesh Mishra, Pankaj Kashyap, Bhavna Sahu

First published in London, United Kingdom, 2021 by IntechOpen
IntechOpen is the global imprint of INTECHOPEN LIMITED, registered in England and Wales, registration number: 11086078, 5 Princes Gate Court, London, SW7 2QJ, United Kingdom
Printed in Croatia

British Library Cataloguing-in-Publication Data
A catalogue record for this book is available from the British Library

Additional hard and PDF copies can be obtained from orders@intechopen.com

Drug Metabolism
Edited by Katherine Dunnington
p. cm.
Print ISBN 978-1-83968-879-9
Online ISBN 978-1-83968-880-5
eBook (PDF) ISBN 978-1-83968-881-2

For EU product safety concerns:
IN TECH d.o.o., Prolaz Marije Krucifikse Kozulić 3, 51000 Rijeka, Croatia, info@intechopen.com or visit our website at intechopen.com.

Meet the editor

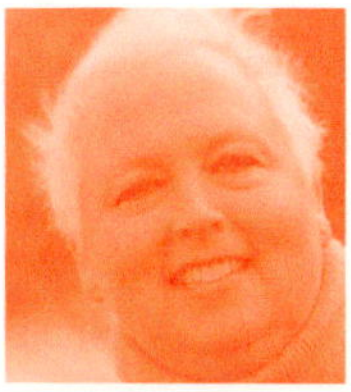

Dr. Katherine "Shelly" Dunnington resides and works in the Midwest United States in the state of Kansas. She is a pharmacokineticist with training in pharmaceutical science and cellular or molecular biology and originally was a practicing pharmacist both in hospital and retail settings. She is currently a senior principal scientist in the Data Management and Biometrics department at Celerion, a pharmaceutical contract research organization. With 21 years in contract research, Dr. Dunnington has many roles in her current position, including training or mentoring scientists; consulting on clinical study design and conduct; analysis, interpretation, and reporting of clinical PK/PD and cardiac safety data; and software validation. Dr. Dunnington holds both a bachelor's degree in pharmacy and an interdisciplinary Ph.D. from the University of Missouri-Kansas City.

Contents

Preface

Drug metabolism comprises the identification, characterization, and quantification of the chemicals or compounds produced in an animal or human upon administration of a drug. Research practices not only require the chemical structure but also aim to determine the pharmacological activities and/or toxicity of these compounds. This is first performed in animals, as studies attempt to identify and quantify metabolites, and later in humans, with care to further characterize metabolites that are either unique to or produced disproportionately in humans compared to animals. Characterization includes the determination of enzyme systems or other biological mechanisms that produce each identified metabolite; this information is used to predict potential drug-drug interactions with other compounds that increase or decrease metabolite formation and sources of biological variability in response or toxicity with varying patient genetics, which affect CYP isoform expression. This book's purpose is to provide a better understanding of the biology and current technology applied in the field of drug metabolism.

Drug Metabolism begins with a review of the various structures and functions of the human liver in the chapter entitled *Hepatocytes and Their Role in Metabolism*. The information covered in this chapter is key to understanding the basic principles involved in the metabolism of drugs at the organ, the cellular, the organelle, and the enzymatic levels. In the chapter *Drug Metabolism in Drug Discovery and Preclinical Development*, the metabolism-related approaches and technology involved before and after the identification of a lead compound are described. This chapter is an up-to-date accounting of how studies relating to drug metabolism are conducted in early drug development.

The second part of the book includes more specialized foci within the realm of drug metabolism. The chapter *From Pharmacogenetics to Gene Expression: Implications for Precision Medicine in Diabetes* examines how drugs and their metabolism are affected by alternate phenotypes among individuals. Furthermore, the chapter *Metabolism of Phytochemicals* is also a description of the highly specialized area of drug metabolism dealing with potential medicinal compounds found in plants. Finally, the chapter In vitro *Metabolic Stability of Drugs and Applications of LC-MS in Metabolite Profiling* is an in-depth look at how liquid chromatography with mass spectrometry detection is applied in quantifying and characterizing potential metabolite species after administration of a drug.

Katherine Dunnington Ph.D.
Celerion,
Data Management and Biometrics Lincoln,
Nebraska, United States

Section 1

Introductory Reviews

Chapter 1

Hepatocytes and Their Role in Metabolism

Shweta Dutta, Saraswati Prasad Mishra, Anil Kumar Sahu, Koushlesh Mishra, Pankaj Kashyap and Bhavna Sahu

Abstract

Liver is one of the vital organ that performs many functions in the human body. Prominently it acts as a metabolizing organ for the body. This chapter elaborately describes hepatocytes along with their morphological features. In addition, it explains the structure of hepatocytes and different parts such as kupffer cells, hepatic stellate and hepatic sinusoids. Moreover present chapter elaborates the varieties of functions that hepatocytes perform such as filtration of blood, acting as a viral incubator, lipophagy and regulation of insulin and glucose. This chapter also explains hepatic injury that is caused by chronic consumption of alcohol along with the mechanism behind it.

Keywords: liver, hepatocytes, kupffer cells, viral incubator, lipophagy

1. Introduction

Liver is one the most vital organ of the human body and it is the largest among all other organs found in humans. There is incomplete separation of liver into lobes. These lobes are covered externally by a thin capsule of connective tissue. Liver is made up of different kinds of cells which interact with one another to perform specified functions. Hepatocytes or hepatic parenchymal cells are approximately 60% of the total cells found in the liver. Hepatocytes hold 80% of total volume of the organ. Hepatocytes are arranged into laminae in such a way that they connect with each other forming a 3 dimensional lattice. The space between the lattices is filled by hepatic sinusoid that performs the function of providing nourishment to the parenchymal cells of the 3 dimensional lattice. Other than the lattice, sinusoids and the non-parenchymal cells form the remaining volume of organ. The different types of non-parenchymal cells found are the inter-luminal kupffer cells, sinusoidal endothelial cell and perisinusoidal stellate cells [1].

When blood passes through the liver the hepatocytes behave as a filter for blood that enters the liver. This behavior of liver helps in production of plasma protein and in endocytic uptake of variety of substances like lipid, trophic agents and growth factors. As liver performs the function of purification and is always in contact of agents like alcohol, excessive fat, pathogens or drugs, it is at higher risk of damage by these agents. This chapter will briefly describe organelles of hepatocytes and the functions they perform in the body. Further the chapter will focus on the function of hepatocytes in metabolism. Moreover it will also explain the mechanism of hepatocyte damage [2].

2. Morphology

The structure of hepatocytes is polyhedral in nature. It contains many faces but generally it is 6 in number. These faces are connected with face of other hepatocytes or in some cases it is in contact with sinusoids. Hepatocytes generally have diameters around 20 to 30 μm. They have a round shaped nucleus in the center of cytoplasm. Approximately 25% of hepatocytes found in an adult human contain two nuclei instead of one. Most of these nuclei contains twice the number of chromosomes than a normal cell; thus are deemed tetraploid. In the nuclei, heterochromatin are scattered. The presence of mitotic hepatocytes is not seen generally in normal conditions. However their number increases in conditions like liver injury or in the process of regeneration. Depending upon the physiological state, the cytoplasm of the hepatic cell varies and is influenced by fat or glycogen depots. In a hepatocyte, as many as 100 mitochondria can be seen. Moreover the number of Golgi apparatus found in a hepatocytes accounts to approximately 50. Each Golgi apparatus are arranged in 3–5 cisterns. These cisterns are located near biliary canaliculi, small canal like structures that collecting the bile secreted by hepatocytes. Peroxisomes found in hepatocytes are in numbers of 200 or 300 which is more than found in normal cells (**Figure 1**, **Table 1**) [3].

2.1 Kupffer cells

Kupffer cells are the macrophages that reside in liver and are the highest number of resident macrophages in body. Kupffer cells are basically phagocytes that remove pathogens that in the circulation. Their presence in hepatic sinusoids allows them to perform the above said function efficiently. They also act against substances which are immunoreactive that enter through the portal circulation from the gastrointestinal tract. As Kupffer cells act against immunoreactive substances that enter from the GIT to portal circulation so they can be regarded as a barrier in the gut. It inhibits many inflammation that may occur due to these immunoreactive substances by destroying them in hepatic sinusoids. The Kupffer cell also plays a major role in clearing the dead red blood cells and comprise the mononuclear phagocytic system due to its phagocytic activity. Though Kupffer cells plays a major role in in protecting the liver from injuries due to alcohol, drugs or toxins, however their

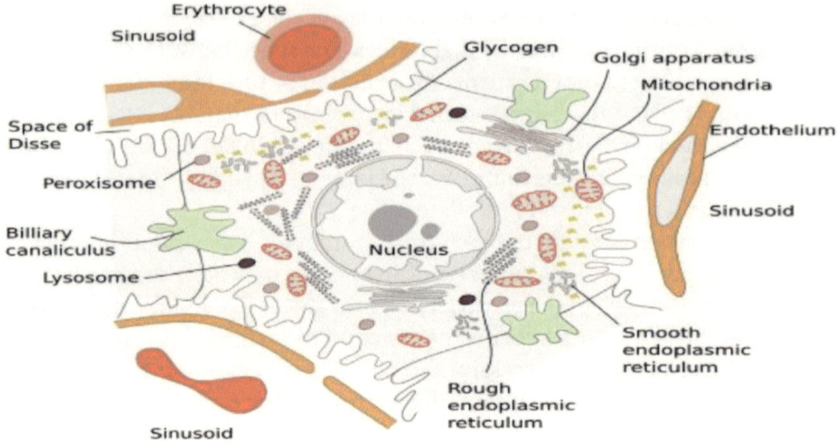

Figure 1.
Hepatocyte ultrastructure [3].

Hepatic cell	Function of the cell
Parenchymal Hepatocytes	Chief cell of the liver, synthesis, storage, degredation of portal substance, metabolism, endocrine and exocrine function.
Non parenchymal cells	
Sinusoidal endothelial cells	Fenestrated plexus allows contact of portal blood with hepatoctyes.
Kupffer cells	Liver phagocytes, release cytokines.
Stellate cell	Injury, precursor to myofibroblast, vitamin A storage.
Cholangiocyte	Transport bile, secrete bicarbonate and water.

Table 1.
Hepatic cell type and their functions [4].

inflammatory response leads to conditions like chronic inflammation in liver which may be due alcoholic as well as non-alcoholic liver disease [5].

2.2 Hepatic sinusoids

The hepatic sinusoids are covered by specific endothelial cells that leads to formation of a barrier, which is porous in nature, that aid in exchange of materials among the hepatocytes and blood. The endothelial cells helps the clusters of differentiation markers such as CD14, CD16, CDw32, CD36, CD54, CD13 and CD4. They possess specific phenotype for portal venules, capillary endothelium, and terminal hepatic venule. It can be seen that the endothelium of portal tract arterioles, branches of portal vein and central veins binds with *U. europaeus* lectin and eventually stains CD34 and CD31 positively [6]. However sinusoidal endothelium in the majority of lobules are generally negative for CD34 and laminin. Positive staining of sinusoids is seen with carcinoma of hepatic cells as they stain sinusoid like vessels [7, 8]. Sinusoidal lumen contains cells such as kupffer cells, macrophages which can be seen by immunostain for CD68. Activated kupffer cells are positive with DPAS and muramidase [9, 10].

2.3 Hepatic stellate cells

Hepatic stellate cells belong to the family of myofibroblasts. Stellate cells show their activity in the process of fibrogenesis and regulate flow of sinusoidal blood [11, 12]. They play the role of antigen presenting cells as well. Stellate cells during the childhood or adolescence phases are positive for actin whereas they are negative in adults and become positive only when there is any pathological condition [13]. Whereas in the case of synaptophysin, which is one of the main synaptic vesicle protein p38 and is encoded by the SYP gene, activated as well as resting stellate cells are positive. Stellate cells normally cannot be seen in a healthy liver whereas in pathological conditions they can be identified by vacuolated cytoplasm and a nucleus that becomes scalloped. Hepatic stellate cells are also related to the synthesis of collagen [14, 15].

3. Function of hepatocytes includes

Hepatic cytochromes P450 enzymes found in hepatocytes are one of the major enzymes that metabolize drugs. Hepatocytes also act a factory for protein and biliary secretion. Moreover hepatocytes also behave as an endocytic blood-filtering machine. Hepatocytes aid in detoxification of blood.

3.1 Hepatic cytochromes P450 involved in drug metabolism

The cytochromes P450 are terminal oxidase that comes under the superfamily of hemoproteins. This super family P450 has around 154 genes that can be seen in case of 23 eukaryotes in both plants and animal along with 6 prokaryotes. Among all the isoform of CYPP450, CYP1, CYP2 and CYP3 are known to play important roles in majority of drug metabolism. P450 are responsible for catalyzing some of the reactions such as hydroxylation, dealkylation, and oxygenation. These cytochromes also have ability to catalyze reductive reactions where the metabolite produced from the reaction leads to inactivation of P450 [16].

Most xenobiotics are eliminated from body after undergoing chemical modification. The process of chemical modification of drug can be referred as biotransformation. In the process of biotransformation, lipophilic drugs are rendered more hydrophilic so that they can be excreted easily. Biotransformation occurs through two phases namely: Phase I and Phase II. Phase I reaction is also termed as functionalization reaction whereas Phase II reaction is called as conjugation reaction. In phase I reactions, the parent compounds undergoes oxidative processes to form more polar metabolites. In some case more reactive metabolites are also produced. The Phase I reactions are broadly of three types namely oxidation, reduction and hydrolysis. In phase II reactions, the parent compound or its Phase I metabolites are conjugated with endogenous substances like sulfate, glutathione or glucuronic acids to from a more water soluble and less toxic product that easily excrete out from the body.

Examples of Phase II reactions are

i. Glucuronide conjugation: Compounds like Paracetamol, aspirin, chloramphenicol that are having carboxyl group or hydroxyl groups are conjugated with glucuronic acids.

ii. Acetylation: occurs in compounds that has either amino or hydrazine in their structure. Examples of such compounds are sulfonamide, clonazepam.

iii. Methylation: is generally seen in compounds like adrenaline, methyldopa or histamine which contain amines or phenols in their structure.

iv. Sulfate conjugation: A phenolic compound also may undergo sulfate conjugation as well.

v. Glycine conjugation: Compounds such as salicylates which contain carboxylic group gets conjugated with glycine.

Metabolism of diverse ranges of xenobiotic are carried out by enzymes such as cytochrome (CYP) and flavin monooxygenases. CYP are found in liver predominantly and are also found in organs like gastrointestinal tract (GIT), lungs and placenta. 16 gene families and 29 sub families of CYP are found in human beings. Among these families, family 1, 2 and 3 are mostly responsible for biotransformation of xenobiotic. Most abundant CYP found in liver of adult humans is CYP3A4. CYP450 are also known to express more than 2000 mutation and ultimately shows polymorphisms. Some of the CYP also shows single nucleotide polymorphism (SNP). Some important polymorphism are seen in 1A2, 2C9, 2C19 and 2D6. The genetic variation seen in the polymorphs are Mendelian inherited and are responsible for the catalytic variation they show in towards xenobiotic. Due to polymorphism, pharmacokinetic as well pharmacodynamics activities of drugs may show variations. When variability is seen in plasma concentration of drugs, it may lead to either toxicity due to exaggerated plasma concentration or suboptimal actions may be seen when plasma concentration is not achieved. If a new drug is metabolized by polymorphic enzyme then it can be considered as a drawback for the new drug because of the variation that can be shown to by the polymorphic enzyme [17, 18].

3.2 The hepatocyte as a protein and biliary secretion factory

Hepatocytes contains many organelles that are secretory in nature as well as many mitochondria. Because of the presence of large number of endoplasmic reticulum and golgi bodies, the secretory activity of hepatocytes get overshadowed. Generally proteins that are secreted from hepatocytes initiates with ribosomal synthesis after which the polypeptide formed get transported into the lumen of endoplasmic reticulum then it reaches the golgi apparatus where secretory vesicles of golgi apparatus encloses the protein and transport it through exocytosis from hepatocytes [19, 20]. The major proteins that are secreted from hepatocytes are namely albumin, fibrinogen, transferrin and clotting factors. Serum proteins are the most prominent proteins secreted by hepatocytes [21–23]. It is important in context of bile production as well as in production of complex molecular soap that contains conjugated bilirubin, bile acids, electrolytes and phospholipids. Bile has a role in emulsification of fats and their digestion in the intestine as well as in removing xenobiotics and waste products that are produced endogenously. Synthesis of bile takes place in hepatocytes and is then transported to the bile canaliculi. Because of osmotic gradient bile moves through ductules and eventually reaches bile duct. During the transit, the bile is further modified by cholangiocytes and ductular epithelial cells [24]. Then bile goes into the gall bladder and it is released into intestine when needed. An amount of approximately 800 ml bile is secreted daily in the gut. The apical surface of hepatocytes because of thier structure, are tolerant to the bile environment. The apical domain also helps in synthesis, transportation and release of bile acids. Transportation is carried out by the ATP-dependent ABC transporter [25]. Transportation of cytotoxins and foreign substances is carried out by the multidrug resistance protein 1 as well as the multidrug and extrusion protein 1. The remaning content of bile like sulfate conjugates and conjugate bilirubin are exported through the bile salt export pump and multidrug resistance related protein 2. Aquaporin types such as aquaporin 0 and aquaporin 8 carry out the transportation of water to bile [26]. Most of the apical membrane protein moves through transcytosis whereas transporters such as the ABC transporter comes either from Golgi apparatus or through subapical endosomes [27, 28]. The sinusoidal surface is made up with basolateral membrane that makes the connection with the portal blood. Sinusoidal surfaces possess receptosr such as tyrosine kinase and trophic receptors. Moreover it also contains ABC transporter that performs the function of retrieving bile acids and other component sof bile from circulating blood. Conjugated bile acids which are water soluble is retrieved by the help of a transporter called sodium taurocholate cotransporter (NTCP) whereas water insoluble bile acids are retrieved with the help of organic anion transporting polypeptides [29, 30].

3.3 The ultimate endocytic blood-filtering machine

Solute transporters perform the task of transporting bile acids whereas the protein that are found in the sinusoidal membrane plays an important role in internalizing essential components from blood through hepatocytes. Liver being the first organ that is in contact with the nutrients that comes to the gastrointestinal tract, it has evolved into a kind of biological filter that filter out unwanted and potentially damaging substances that could reach those organs which do not have the ability to detoxify them. Liver cells, by the process of endocytosis, internalize materials that are present in extracellular matrix. There are many endocytic mechanisms found in the hepatocytes such as the fluid-phase endocytic mechanism as well as caveolae-based endocytosis. However the most prominent endocytic mechanism is receptor mediated endocytosis (RME) [31, 32]. Hepatocytes are remarkably capable of RME. In the process of RME, basolateral plasma membrane binds with extracellular ligands that present in blood plasma followed by incorporation via clathrin coated pits. When they enter the cell the receptor, ligand and the carrier protein are transported to a different destination within the cell, and are then recycled back and finally degraded by the action of lysosomes and endosomes. Trafficking of endocytic vesicles are controlled by Rab GTPases. Rab GTPase is an enzyme which assists in regulating various steps in membrane trafficking, such as vesicle formation, vesicle movement along actin and tubulin networks, and membrane fusion. Which basically selects specific protein for binding [33, 34]. Rab effector also performs other functions such as vesicle fusion and remodeling of membrane. Uponn ligand stimulation, internalization of half of the insulin along with EGF receptors through clathrin coated pits takes place within one minute [35]. Due to this great ability of endocytosis, hepatocytes are capable of performing the task of filtering blood which enters the hepatic portal system [36].

3.4 Regulation of systemic insulin and glucose

After a meal, pancreatic β-cells secrete insulin in a pulsated manner. Insulin, by binding with insulin receptors, initiates the utilization of dietary glucose as well as its storage in the adipose tissue, muscles and in liver. Liver plays a major role in maintaining the homeostasis of glucose in the body. Hepatocyte stores around 100 g in glycogen polysaccharides [37, 38]. Postprandial release of insulin causes a decline in the blood glucose level. However to counteract this effect glucagon, a hormone that is secreted by pancreatic α cells stimulate the utilization of glucose through the cyclic AMP- protein kinase A (cAMP–PKA) pathway [39, 40]. Through RME hepatocytes clear around 80% of blood insulin before it reaches peripheral tissue [41]. The phosphatidylinositol 3-kinase- protein kinase B (PI3K–AKT) pathway initiates the storage of lipid and glucose. Whereas activation of the said pathway depends upon the endocytic uptake of insulin receptor [42]. When endocytosis of the insulin receptor takes place, it leads to dissociation of insulin ligand inside the endosomes and sorting of insulin receptors is done and through recycling pathway as they are trafficed back to the plasma membrane [43].

3.5 Endocytosis of two types of transferrin receptors (TfRs) is key for iron homeostasis

One of the essential functions that is performed by liver is maintaining systemic iron homeostasis. Iron is a vital component in processes like cellular function, gene transcription, DNA replication and mitochondrial respiration [44, 45]. The human body depends on the dietary sources to fulfill its iron requirements as it is not produced in the body itself. This iron gets stored in the liver cells and macrophages [46]. There are two different endocytosis mechanisms through which iron storage and release takes place. Within the circulation, iron gets circulated by combining with a protein called as transferrin. Transferrin acts a ligand for the transferrin receptors (TfRs). There are two types of transferrin receptors namely TfR1 and TfR2 which are found in different tissues and play a major role in homeostasis of iron [44, 45, 47]. TfR1 is abundantly expressed in the body and these receptors are concerned with iron uptake into the cells. Whereas TfR2 are found in erythroid cells and hepatocytes. These receptors aid in sensing of the presence or absence of iron in the human body and eventually helps in maintaining the homeostasis of iron [48]. Iron transferrin complex binds to the transferrin receptor and through a clathrin-mediated endocytosis process is internalized. Afterward the complex dissociatea inside the cell and transferrins along with TfR receptor are transported back to the cell membrane [49]. The iron that remains in the endosome is transported to the cytoplasm with by a transporter called DMT1. In the cytoplasm iron complexes with another protein called ferritin. The Mmajority of the ferritin stays in hepatocytes and sequesters around 4000 atoms of iron, making them available to structures of sub-cellular level such as DNA [50]. Moreover, hepatocytes also regulate iron release into the circulation by stimulating cells which are rich in iron stores such as macrophages and Kupffer cells [51]. TfR2 which is responsible to sense the level of iron in circulation stimulate the release a peptide called as hepcidin from liver cells whenever iron levels exceed normal. Hepcidin binds with ferroportin, an export transporter of iron [52, 53]. Hepcidin initiates ferroportin degradation in the endosomes by stimulating endocytosis and eventually reduces the export of iron and promotes its storage [54]. Hepatocytes are different from other epithelial cells as they participate in the internalization of iron through TfR1 and maintain homeostasis of with TfR2.

3.6 Lipoproteins, lipid droplets (LDs), lipolysis, and lipophagy

The liver plays an important role in metabolism of lipid. Liver act as a depot for storage of lipid that are taken up from circulation. Breakdown and release of the stored lipid also takes place through liver. Dietary lipids are taken up by the liver cells as chylomicron remnants, although a significant amount of the lipid is released back into the blood in the form of very low-density lipoprotein (VLDL). Assembly of VLDL and translation and translocation of protein apoB100 inside the rough endoplasmic reticulum lumen occur simulateneously and binds to various neutral lipids. The lipoproteins which are secreted deliver lipid to tissues such as muscle or adipose either for storage or for utilization as an energy source. Hepatocytes clear 80–90% of these lipids from the blood stream [55]. Internalization of lipoproteins present in plasma into clathrin-coated vesicles is done by hepatocytes by the process of RME [56]. LDLR is the low-density lipoprotein receptor which helps lipoprotein-borne cholesterol enter into cells. LDLR identifies the surface proteins such as ApoE and ApoB100 present on low density lipoproteins and act as a station for retrieval of circulating lipids [57]. Conditions which affect the process of endocytosis of lipoprotein hugely impacts the level of cholesterols in the circulation and are the major reason for disease associated with heart and blood vessels [58]. Cholesterols, in the form HDL, also come back to the liver from macrophages that are present in artery as well as from peripheral tissues by a process called reverse cholesterol transport. Hepatocytes also takes up enterocyte-derived chylomicrons which contains retinyl esters (REs). Very small amounts of RE is taken up by hepatocytes for storage whereas maximum amounts are transported to hepatic stellate cells [59–61]. In endoplasmic reticulum lipid droplets (LDs) biosynthesis takes place leading to distention of neutral membrane lipids to cytoplasm [62]. Liver contains different types of lipolytic enzymes. These lipolytic enzymes, adipose triglyceride lipase (ATGL) and this family of enzymes act as catalyst in lipolysis of triglycerides and catabolism of LDs present in cytoplasm [63]. Moreover carboxylesterases perform the task of mobilizing triglycerol (TAG) from hepatic cells and mediate distribution of stored fatty acids from LDs present in cytoplasm to VLDL which are formed in endoplasmic reticulum [64, 65]. This process of autophagy also is critical in LDs turnover. Lipophagy is a process where LDs are engulfed by hepatic autophagic membrane to form autophagosomes, then by the action of autolysosomes, LDs are broken down with by acidic lipase and hydrolases [66].

3.7 The hepatocyte as a viral incubator

Liver being one the most vascular metabolizing organs, a large amount of blood enters is filtered. However, as liver receives such a huge amount of blood, it is always exposed to variety pathogens such as bacteria, virus or fungus. To counteract these pathogens hepatocytes release proteins, which in turn lead to stimulation of an innate immune response [67]. However some of the viruses by pass this defense mechanism of liver and enter the hepatocytes. Hepatitis B virus (HBV) and hepatitis C virus C (HCV) are viruses that enter hepatocytes. Infection caused by either these two can lead to severe liver disease [68]. HBV is a DNA virus and belongs to the family of Hepadnaviridae, it enters hepatic cells through a receptor called Na + taurocholate cotransporting polypeptide (NTCP) which is present on the surface of sinusoidal plasma membrane [69]. HBV is taken into hepatocytes by the process of endocytosis whereas there is no concrete idea about their escape [70]. According to studies, HBV replicates and releases infectious particles by hijacking the vesicular components such as multivesicular endosomes and autophagosomes [71]. Viral genomes enter the nucleus to undergo transcription, where the pregenomic RNA gets to cytosol and undergoes the process of reverse transcription and packs the resultant DNA into icosahedral nucleocapsid [72]. HBV then utilizes the secretary ability of the liver cells to release mature viruses into the circulation.

HCV is an RNA virus which belongs to Flaviviridae family. It enters hepatocytes by posing itself as a lipoprotein particle. Mature virus expresses two kind of apolipoproteins namely E1 and E2 on their surface that eventually leads to binding to receptors such as LDLR and CD81, which are found in sinusoidal membrane of hepatocytes, leading to internalization of virus by the process of RME [73]. Then the virus fuses with endosomes. Finally the RNA genome which freely acts as a template for synthesizing structural and nonstructural proteins of HCV. The core capsid and nonstructural protein namely NS5A promotes the assembly of nascent HCV near the endoplasmic reticulum [74]. Once they are assembled the mature virus particles are secreted out of the hepatocytes [75].

4. Hepatocyte injury

Alcohol is known to cause hepatic injury but it is the metabolite of alcohol that is produced during metabolism which is hepatotoxic. In the initial stage of alcoholic liver disease, steatosis occurs; whereas in case of acute or chronic exposure to alcohol leads to accumulation of triglycerides as well as enhances the expression of lipogenic enzyme. Moreover, the enzymes which are responsible for fatty acid oxidation are down regulated [76]. Advanced stages of alcoholic liver disease are associated with conditions like fibrosis and cirrhosis. In hepatic fibrosis extracellular matrix protein gets deposited and forms scars such as those that occur in cutaneous wounds [77, 78].

4.1 Mechanisms of hepatocyte injury by excess alcohol consumption

Hepatocytes are the site of alcohol metabolism. Metabolites of alcohol that are produced during its metabolism are the major reason of hepatic injury. Chronic consumption of alcohol is major risk factor for hepatic injury. In reversible alcoholic liver disease, hepatocyte shows a condition called as steatosis where accumulation of cytoplasmic LDs have accumulated. Whereas in acute or chronic stages of liver disease triglycerides accumulate because of enhanced expression of lipogenic enzymes as well as down regulation of those enzymes which are concerned in oxidation of fatty acid. Moreover LD metabolism, specifically its catabolism, is hampered due to impaired lipophagy [79]. Additionally lipolysis is impaired through cytoplasmic lipases [80]. Fibrosis and cirrhosis are the characteristics seen in later stages of alcoholic liver disease. In the process of alcohol metabolism, alcohol isconverted to acetaldehyde in the presence of an enzyme called alcohol dehydrogenase present in the cytosol. Acetaldehyde is converted to acetate in mitochondria. The acetate produced is utilized in the citric acid cycle for the formation of acetyl-CoA. For alcohol metabolism, co factor NAD+ is required in large amount, so it is depleted and in turn the reduction –oxidation (redox) state of ethanol exposed hepatocytes isaltered. This leads to dysregulation of carbohydrate and lipid metabolism as well as inhibition of NAD+ dependent enzymes that are responsible prevention of hepatic injury [81]. Cytochrome P450 2E1 (CYP2E1) also metabolizes alcohol, in addition to alcohol dehydrogenase, and produces acetaldehyde along with highly reactive oxygen and hydroxyethyl radicals. These metabolites are capable of forming bonds with protein, DNA and lipids [82]. CYP2E1 also produces oxidative stress which is one of the major causes of alcohol induced hepatic dysfunction. Eventually oxidative stress leads to endoplasmic reticulum stress resulting in apoptosis of the hepatic cell, steatosis and inflammation due to build up of unfolded protein [83]. Moreover alcohol induces an increase in mitochondrial permeability leading to alteration in homeostasis of cellular energy and eventually apoptosis in addition to generation of reactive oxygen species [84]. These acetaldehyde and oxygen radicals are the major mechanism of liver injury as they stimulate hepatic dysfunction and inflammatory response [85]. Consumption of alcohol induces production of enzyme CYP2E1 and it reinforces this cycle of hepatic damage again.

5. Conclusion and future perspectives

This chapter it illustrates that hepatocytes have the unique ability to perform a variety of functions. It can be called a jack of all trades. Hepatocytes perform the task of detoxification of blood in one hand and also does the packaging and secretion of components such as lipid, protein and bile. In addition they take up nutrients from the blood stream. However, if there is any kind of compromise in the functioning of liver related to membrane trafficking it can lead to many diseases like cirrhosis, hepatitis, fibrosis and even carcinoma of the liver. The present chapter elaborated on the functioning of liver and the associated condition of liver when there is a variety malfunctions. Liver being the major organ in metabolism as well as in detoxification of blood and nutrient uptake, through a series of detailed future research on its function and effect of various pathogenic conditions on its functioning can be accurately estimated. This chapter concludes that an accurate estimate will eventually be a boon to develop better treatment of the disease conditions associated liver.

Author details

Shweta Dutta[1*], Saraswati Prasad Mishra[2], Anil Kumar Sahu[1], Koushlesh Mishra[3], Pankaj Kashyap[1] and Bhavna Sahu[2]

1 Royal College of Pharmacy, Raipur, Chhattisgarh, India

2 RITEE College of Pharmacy, Raipur, Chhattisgarh, India

3 Raigarh College of Pharmacy, Raigarh, Chhattisgarh, India

*Address all correspondence to: shweta.run46@gmail.com

References

[1] McCuskey R. Anatomy of the liver. Zakim and Boyer's Hepatology: a textbook of liver disease. 2012; 6: 3-19.

[2] Schulze RJ, Schott MB, Casey CA, Tuma PL, McNiven MA. The cell biology of the hepatocyte: A membrane trafficking machine. Journal of Cell Biology. 2019 Jul 1; 218(7): 2096-2112.

[3] Leeuwenhoek A. Atlas of plant and animal histology 2021

[4] Juza RM, Pauli EM. Clinical and surgical anatomy of the liver: a review for clinicians. Clinical Anatomy. 2014 Jul;27(5):764-769

[5] Naito M, Hasegawa G, Ebe Y, Yamamoto T. Differentiation and function of Kupffer cells. Medical Electron Microscopy. 2004 Mar 1;37(1):16-28.

[6] Dhillon AP, Colombari R, Savage K, et al. An immunohistochemical study of the blood vessels within primary hepatocellular tumours. Liver. 1992;12:311-318

[7] Shafizadeh N, Kakar S. Diagnosis of welldifferentiated hepatocellular lesions: role of immunohistochemistry and other ancillary techniques. Adv Anat Pathol. 2011;18:438-445.

[8] Matsukuma S, Takeo H, Utsumi Y, et al. In hepatic venous outflow obstruction, alcoholic liver disease, and nonalcoholic fatty liver disease, centrilobular scars, CD34+ vessels, and keratin 7+ hepatocytes are in close proximity. Virchows Arch. 2017;470:411-420.

[9] Norris S, Collins C, Doherty DG, et al. Resident human hepatic lymphocytes are phenotypically different from circulating lymphocytes. J Hepatol. 1998;28:84-90.

[10] Nakatani K, Kaneda K, Seki S, et al. Pit cells as liver-associated natural killer cells: morphology and function. Med Electron Microsc. 2004;37:29-36.

[11] Pinzani M. Hepatic stellate (Ito) cells: expanding roles for a liver-specific pericyte. J Hepatol. 1995;22:700-706.

[12] Rockey DC. Hepatic blood flow regulation by stellate cells in normal and injured liver. Semin Liver Dis. 2001;21:337-349.

[13] Schmitt-Graff A, Kruger S, Bochard F, et al. Modulation of alpha smooth muscle actin and desmin expression in perisinusoidal cells of normal and diseased human livers. Am J Pathol. 1991;138:1233-1242.

[14] Cassiman D, Roskams T. Beauty is in the eye of the beholder: emerging concepts and pitfalls in hepatic stellate cell research. Hepatol. 2002;37:527-535.

[15] Ramadori G, Saile B. Mesenchymal cell in the liver: one cell type or two? Liver. 2002;22:283-294.

[16] Wrighton SA, Stevens JC. The human hepatic cytochromes P450 involved in drug metabolism. Critical reviews in toxicology. 1992 Jan 1;22(1):1-21

[17] Donato MT, Castell JV. Strategies and molecular probes to investigate the role of cytochrome P450 in drug metabolism. Clinical Pharmacokinetics. 2003 Feb;42(2):153-178.

[18] De Montellano PR, editor. Cytochrome P450: structure, mechanism, and biochemistry. Springer Science & Business Media; 2005.

[19] Rapoport, T.A., L. Li, and E. Park. 2017. Structural and Mechanistic Insights into Protein Translocation. Annu. Rev. Cell Dev. Biol. 33:369-390.

doi: 10.1146/annurev-cellbio-100616-060439

[20] Saucan L and Palade GE, 1994 Membrane and secretory proteins are transported from the Golgi complex to the sinusoidal plasmalemma of hepatocytes by distinct vesicular carriers. J. Cell Biol. 125:733-741. https://doi.org/10.1083/jcb.125.4.733)

[21] Peters, T. 1996. All about albumin: biochemistry, genetics, and medical applications. Academic Press, San Diego.

[22] Arroyo, V., R. García-Martinez, and X. Salvatella. 2014. Human serum albumin, systemic inflammation, and cirrhosis. J. Hepatol. 61:396-407. https://doi.org/10.1016/j.jhep.2014.04.012

[23] Levitt, D.G., and M.D. Levitt. 2016. Human serum albumin homeostasis: a new look at the roles of synthesis, catabolism, renal and gastrointestinal excretion, and the clinical value of serum albumin measurements. Int. J. Gen. Med. 9:229-255. https://doi.org/10.2147/IJGM.S102819

[24] Banales, J.M., R.C. Huebert, T. Karlsen, M. Strazzabosco, N.F. LaRusso, and G.J. Gores. 2019. Cholangiocyte pathobiology. Nat. Rev. Gastroenterol. Hepatol. 16:269-281. https://doi.org/10.1038/s41575-019-0125-y

[25] Boyer, J.L. 2013. Bile formation and secretion. Compr. Physiol. 3:1035-1078. (for an extensive list, see Boyer, 2013).

[26] Marinelli, R.A., P.S. Tietz, A.J. Caride, B.Q. Huang, and N.F. LaRusso. 2003. Water transporting properties of hepatocyte basolateral and canalicular plasma membrane domains. J. Biol. Chem. 278:43157-43162. 10.1074/jbc.M305899200

[27] Kipp, H., and I.M. Arias. 2000. Newly synthesized canalicular ABC transporters are directly targeted from the Golgi to the hepatocyte apical domain in rat liver. J. Biol. Chem. 275:15917-15925. https://doi.org/10.1074/jbc.M909875199

[28] Zeigerer, A., J. Gilleron, R.L. Bogorad, G. Marsico, H. Nonaka, S. Seifert, H. Epstein-Barash, S. Kuchimanchi, C.G. Peng, V.M. Ruda, et al. 2012. Rab5 is necessary for the biogenesis of the endolysosomal system in vivo. Nature. 485:465-470. https://doi.org/10.1038/nature11133

[29] Ihrke, G., and A.L. Hubbard. 1995. Control of vesicle traffic in hepatocytes. Prog. Liver Dis 13:3-99.

[30] Tuma, P.L., and A.L. Hubbard. 2001. The hepatocyte surface: dynamic polarity. In The Liver: Biology and Pathobiology. I.M. Arias, J.L. Boyer, F.V. Chisari, N. Fausto, D. Schachter, and D.A. Shafritz, editors. Lippincott Williams and Wilkins, Philadelphia, PA.

[31] Mayor, S., R.G. Parton, and J.G. Donaldson. 2014. Clathrin-independent pathways of endocytosis. Cold Spring Harb. Perspect. Biol. 6:a016758. https://doi.org/10.1101/cshperspect.a016758

[32] Kaksonen, M., and A. Roux. 2018. Mechanisms of clathrin-mediated endocytosis. Nat. Rev. Mol. Cell Biol. 19:313-326. https://doi.org/10.1038/nrm.2017.132

[33] Zhen, Y., and H. Stenmark. 2015. Cellular functions of Rab GTPases at a glance. J. Cell Sci. 128:3171-3176. https://doi.org/10.1242/jcs.166074

[34] Pfeffer, S.R. 2017. Rab GTPases: master regulators that establish the secretory and endocytic pathways. Mol. Biol. Cell. 28:712-715. https://doi.org/10.1091/mbc.e16-10-0737

[35] Burgess, J.W., A.P. Bevan, J.J. Bergeron, and B.I. Posner. 1992. Pharmacological doses of insulin equalize insulin receptor

phosphotyrosine content but not tyrosine kinase activity in plasmalemmal and endosomal membranes. Biochem. Cell Biol. 70:1151-1158. https://doi.org/10.1139/o92

[36] Di Guglielmo, G.M., P.C. Baass, W.J. Ou, B.I. Posner, and J.J. Bergeron. 1994. Compartmentalization of SHC, GRB2 and mSOS, and hyperphosphorylation of Raf-1 by EGF but not insulin in liver parenchyma. EMBO J. 13:4269-4277. https://doi.org/10.1002/j.1460-2075.1994.tb06747.x

[37] Tokarz, V.L., P.E. MacDonald, and A. Klip. 2018. The cell biology of systemic insulin function. J. Cell Biol. 217:2273-2289. https://doi.org/10.1083/jcb.201802095

[38] Wasserman, D.H. 2009. Four grams of glucose. Am. J. Physiol. Endocrinol. Metab. 296:E11–E21. https://doi.org/10.1152/ajpendo.90563

[39] Authier, F., and B. Desbuquois. 2008. Glucagon receptors. Cell. Mol. Life Sci. 65:1880-1899. https://doi.org/10.1007/s00018-008-7479-6

[40] Habegger, K.M., K.M. Heppner, N. Geary, T.J. Bartness, R. DiMarchi, and M.H. Tsch¨op. 2010. The metabolic actions of glucagon revisited. Nat. Rev. Endocrinol. 6:689-697. https://doi.org/10.1038/nrendo.2010.

[41] Meier, J.J., J.D. Veldhuis, and P.C. Butler. 2005. Pulsatile insulin secretion dictates systemic insulin delivery by regulating hepatic insulin extraction in humans. Diabetes. 54:1649-1656. https://doi.org/10.2337/diabetes.54.6.1649

[42] Braccini, L., E. Ciraolo, C.C. Campa, A. Perino, D.L. Longo, G. Tibolla, M. Pregnolato, Y. Cao, B. Tassone, F. Damilano, et al. 2015. PI3K-C2γ is a Rab5 effector selectively controlling endosomal Akt2 activation downstream of insulin signalling. Nat. Commun. 6:7400. https://doi.org/10.1038/ncomms8400.

[43] Fehlmann, M., J.L. Carpentier, E. Van Obberghen, P. Freychet, P. Thamm, D. Saunders, D. Brandenburg, and L. Orci. 1982. Internalized insulin receptors are recycled to the cell surface in rat hepatocytes. Proc. Natl. Acad. Sci. USA. 79:5921-5925. https://doi.org/10.1073/pnas.79.19.5921

[44] Ganz, T. 2013. Systemic iron homeostasisPhysiol. Rev. 93:1721-1741. doi: 10.1152/physrev.00008.2013

[45] Bogdan, A.R., M. Miyazawa, K. Hashimoto, and Y. Tsuji. 2016. Regulators of Iron Homeostasis: New Players in Metabolism, Cell Death, and Disease. Trends Biochem. Sci. 41:274-286. https://doi.org/10.1016/j.tibs.2015.11.012

[46] Rishi, G., and V.N. Subramaniam. 2017. The liver in regulation of iron homeostasis. Am. J. Physiol. Gastrointest. Liver Physiol. 313:G157–G165. https://doi.org/10.1152/ajpgi.00004.2017

[47] Kawabata, H. 2019. Transferrin and transferrin receptors update. Free Radic. Biol. Med. 133:46-54. https://doi.org/10.1016/j.freeradbiomed.2018.06.037

[48] West, A.P. Jr., M.J. Bennett, V.M. Sellers, N.C. Andrews, C.A. Enns, and P.J. Bjorkman. 2000. Comparison of the interactions of transferrin receptor and transferrin receptor 2 with transferrin and the hereditary hemochromatosis protein HFE. J. Biol. Chem. 275:38135-38138. 10.1074/jbc.C000664200

[49] Schroeder, B., and M.A. McNiven. 2014. Importance of endocytic pathways in liver function and disease. Compr. Physiol. 4:1403-1417. 10.1002/cphy.c140001

[50] Theil, E.C. 1987. Ferritin: structure, gene regulation, and cellular function in animals, plants, and microorganisms. Annu. Rev. Biochem. 56:289-315. https://doi.org/10.1146/annurev.bi.56.070187.001445

[51] Wallace, D.F., L. Summerville, and V.N. Subramaniam. 2007. Targeted disruption of the hepatic transferrin receptor 2 gene in mice leads to iron overload. Gastroenterology. 132:301-310. https://doi.org/10.1053/j.gastro.2006.11.028

[52] Nemeth, E., M.S. Tuttle, J. Powelson, M.B. Vaughn, A. Donovan, D.M. Ward, T. Ganz, and J. Kaplan. 2004. Hepcidin regulates cellular iron efflux by binding to ferroportin and inducing its internalization. Science. 306: 2090-2093. https://doi.org/10.1126/science.1104742

[53] Ramey, G., J.C. Deschemin, B. Durel, F. Canonne-Hergaux, G. Nicolas, and S. Vaulont. 2010. Hepcidin targets ferroportin for degradation in hepatocytes. Haematologica. 95:501-504. https://doi.org/10.3324/haematol.2009.014399

[54] Anderson, G.J., and D.M. Frazer. 2017. Current understanding of iron homeostasis. Am. J. Clin. Nutr. 106(Suppl 6):1559S–1566S. 10.3945/ajcn.117.155804

[55] Spady, D.K. 1992. Hepatic clearance of plasma low density lipoproteins. Semin. Liver Dis. 12:373-385. https://doi.org/10.1055/s-2008-1040407

[56] Zanoni, P., S. Velagapudi, M. Yalcinkaya, L. Rohrer, and A. von Eckardstein. 2018. Endocytosis of lipoproteins. Atherosclerosis. 275:273-295. doi: 10.1016/j.atherosclerosis.2018.06.881

[57] Goldstein, J.L., and M.S. Brown. 2009. The LDL receptor. Arterioscler. Thromb. Vasc. Biol. 29:431-438. https://doi.org/10.1161/ATVBAHA.108.179564

[58] Defesche, J.C., S.S. Gidding, M. Harada-Shiba, R.A. Hegele, R.D. Santos, and A.S. Wierzbicki. 2017. Familial hypercholesterolaemia. Nat. Rev. Dis. Primers. 3:17093. https://doi.org/10.1038/nrdp.2017.93

[59] Friedman, S.L. 2008. Hepatic stellate cells: protean, multifunctional, and enigmatic cells of the liver. Physiol. Rev. 88:125-172. https://doi.org/10.1152/physrev.00013.2007

[60] Blaner, W.S. 2019. Vitamin A signaling and homeostasis in obesity, diabetes, and metabolic disorders. Pharmacol. Ther. 197:153-178. 10.1016/j.pharmthera.2019.01.006

[61] Blaner, W.S., S.M. O'Byrne, N. Wongsiriroj, J. Kluwe, D.M. D'Ambrosio, H. Jiang, R.F. Schwabe, E.M. Hillman, R. Piantedosi, and J. Libien. 2009. Hepatic stellate cell lipid droplets: a specialized lipid droplet for retinoid storage. Biochim. Biophys. Acta. 1791:467-473. 10.1016/j.bbalip.2008.11.001

[62] Walther, T.C., J. Chung, and R.V. Farese Jr. 2017. Lipid Droplet Biogenesis. Annu. Rev. Cell Dev. Biol. 33:491-510. https://doi.org/10.1146/annurev cellbio-100616-060608

[63] Kienesberger, P.C., M. Oberer, A. Lass, and R. Zechner. 2009. Mammalian patatin domain containing proteins: a family with diverse lipolytic activities involved in multiple biological functions. J. Lipid Res. 50: S63–S68. https://doi.org/10.1194/jlr.R800082-JLR200

[64] Gilham, D., M. Alam, W. Gao, D.E. Vance, and R. Lehner. 2005. Triacylglycerol hydrolase is localized to the endoplasmic reticulum by an unusual retrieval sequence where it participates in VLDL assembly without utilizing VLDL lipids as substrates. Mol. Biol. Cell. 16:984-996. doi.org/10.1091/mbc.e04-03-0224

[65] Lian, J., R. Nelson, and R. Lehner. 2018. Carboxylesterases in lipid metabolism: from mouse to human. Protein Cell. 9:178-195. 10.1007/s13238-017-0437-z

[66] Moretti, F., P. Bergman, S. Dodgson, D. Marcellin, I. Claerr, J.M. Goodwin, R. DeJesus, Z. Kang, C. Antczak, D. Begue, et al. 2018. TMEM41B is a novel regulator of autophagy and lipid mobilization. EMBO Rep. 19:e45889. https://doi.org/10.15252/embr.201845889

[67] Zhou, Z., M.J. Xu, and B. Gao. 2016. Hepatocytes: a key cell type for innate immunity. Cell. Mol. Immunol. 13:301-315. https://doi.org/10.1038/cmi.2015.97

[68] Stanaway, J.D., A.D. Flaxman, M. Naghavi, C. Fitzmaurice, T. Vos, I. Abubakar, L.J. Abu-Raddad, R. Assadi, N. Bhala, B. Cowie, et al. 2016. The global burden of viral hepatitis from 1990 to 2013: findings from the Global Burden of Disease Study 2013. Lancet. 388:1081-1088. 10.1016/S0140-6736(16)30579-7

[69] Yan,H., G. Zhong, G. Xu,W.He, Z. Jing, Z.Gao, Y.Huang, Y.Qi, B. Peng,H. Wang, et al. 2012. Sodium taurocholate cotransporting polypeptide is a functional receptor for human hepatitis B and D virus. eLife. 1: e00049

[70] Yuen, M.F., D.S. Chen, G.M. Dusheiko, H.L.A. Janssen, D.T.Y. Lau, S.A. Locarnini, M.G. Peters, and C.L. Lai. 2018. Hepatitis B virus infection. Nat. Rev. Dis. Primers. 4:18035. https://doi.org/10.1038/nrdp.2018.35

[71] Sir, D., Y. Tian, W.L. Chen, D.K. Ann, T.S. Yen, and J.H. Ou. 2010. The early autophagic pathway is activated by hepatitis B virus and required for viral DNA replication. Proc. Natl. Acad. Sci. USA. 107:4383-4388. 10.1073/pnas.0911373107

[72] Venkatakrishnan, B., and A. Zlotnick. 2016. The Structural Biology of Hepatitis B Virus: Form and Function. Annul. Rev. Virol 3:429-451. doi.org/10.1146/annurev-virology-110615-042238

[73] Manns, M.P., M. Buti, E. Gane, J.M. Pawlotsky, H. Razavi, N. Terrault, and Z. Younossi. 2017. Hepatitis C virus infection. Nat. Rev. Dis. Primers. 3: 17006. https://doi.org/10.1038/nrdp.2017.

[74] Miyanari, Y., K. Atsuzawa, N. Usuda, K. Watashi, T. Hishiki, M. Zayas, R. Bartenschlager, T. Wakita, M. Hijikata, and K. Shimotohno. 2007. The lipid droplet is an important organelle for hepatitis C virus production. Nat. Cell Biol. 9:1089-1097. https://doi.org/10.1038/ncb1631

[75] Jones, D.M., and J.McLauchlan. 2010. Hepatitis C virus: assembly and release of virus particles. J. Biol. Chem. 285:22733-22739. 10.1074/jbc.R110.133017

[76] Donohue, T.M. Jr. 2007. Alcohol-induced steatosis in liver cells. World J. Gastroenterol. 13:4974-4978. https://doi.org/10.3748/wjg.v13.i37.4974

[77] Seki, E., and R.F. Schwabe. 2015. Hepatic inflammation and fibrosis: functional links and key pathways. Hepatology. 61:1066-1079. 10.1002/hep.27332

[78] Tsuchida, T., and S.L. Friedman. 2017. Mechanisms of hepatic stellate cell activation. Nat. Rev. Gastroenterol. Hepatol. 14:397-411. 10.1038/nrgastro.2017.38

[79] Rasineni, K., B.L. McVicker, D.J. Tuma, M.A. McNiven, and C.A. Casey. 2014. Rab GTPases associate with isolated lipid droplets (LDs) and show altered content after ethanol administration: potential role in alcoholimpaired LD metabolism. Alcohol. Clin. Exp. Res. 38:327-335. doi.org/10.1111/acer.12271

[80] Schott, M.B., K. Rasineni, S.G. Weller, R.J. Schulze, A.C. Sletten, C.A. Casey, and M.A. McNiven. 2017. β-Adrenergic induction of lipolysis in hepatocytes is inhibited by ethanol exposure. J. Biol. Chem. 292:11815-11828. https://doi.org/10.1074/jbc.M117.777748

[81] Tsukamoto, H., and S.C. Lu. 2001. Current concepts in the pathogenesis of alcoholic liver injury. FASEB J. 15:1335-1349. 10.1096/fj.00-0650rev

[82] Tuma, D.J., and C.A. Casey. 2003. Dangerous byproducts of alcohol breakdown-- focus on adducts. Alcohol Res. Health. 27:285-290.

[83] Ji, C. 2015. Advances and New Concepts in Alcohol-Induced Organelle Stress, Unfolded Protein Responses and Organ Damage. Biomolecules. 5: 1099-1121. https://doi.org/10.3390/biom5021099

[84] Das, S.K., and D.M. Vasudevan. 2007. Alcohol-induced oxidative stress. Life Sci. 81:177-187. https://doi.org/10.1016/j.lfs.2007.05.005

[85] Tuma, D.J. 2002. Role of malondialdehyde-acetaldehyde adducts in liver injury. Free Radic Biol Med. 32:303-308. 10.1016/S0891-5849(01)00742-0

Chapter 2

Drug Metabolism in Drug Discovery and Preclinical Development

Benjamin Mann, Roger Melton and David Thompson

Abstract

Drug metabolism or more generally, xenobiotic metabolism, is the biotransformation of exogenous compounds by living organisms, usually through specialized enzymatic systems. The metabolism of experimental therapeutics is an important aspect of pharmacology and translational medicine as the rate and the interindividual variability of drug metabolism can determine the duration and/or efficacy of a drug's pharmacologic action. Since the introduction of metabolites in safety testing guidance by the Food and Drug Administration, major changes have occurred in the experimental methods for the identification and quantification of metabolites, evaluation of metabolites, and the timing of critical nonclinical studies to generate this information.

Keywords: Drug Metabolism, Drug Discovery, Preclinical Development, Lead Selection, Lead Optimization, Drug Candidate Selection, Metabolite Safety Testing, CYP450 Inhibition, CYP450 Induction, Soft Spot Analysis, Metabolite Profiling, Membrane Drug Transporters

1. Introduction

Drug metabolism is a drug-clearing event from systemic circulation influencing efficacy and toxicity in humans and preclinical species. The primary endpoints of enzymatic metabolism studies in both the drug discovery and preclinical stages are to resolve metabolic stability, identify and quantify primary metabolites, identify metabolic routes, and measure the potential for drug–drug interactions (DDI) [1]. The majority of *in vivo* and *in vitro* drug metabolism assessments center around hepatic models as the liver is the main metabolizing organ; however, drug metabolism does occur in other organs and tissues (e.g., lungs, kidneys, and intestine). As a result, drug discovery and preclinical development investigations include evaluation of drug metabolism in both hepatic and extra-hepatic models.

Over the past several decades *in vitro* and *in vivo* methodologies to quantitatively measure the absorption, distribution, metabolism, and excretion (ADME) properties of a chemical entity have matured to the point to where these properties can be reliably modeled and simulated in order to predict the general disposition of the chemical entity (or class of molecules) across multiple species and into humans [2]. As a result, approximations of oral bioavailability (F), total systemic clearance (CL), volume of distribution (Vd), and half-life ($t_{1/2}$) can be predicted and subsequently evaluated. These intrinsic properties of the chemical entity with consideration of the physiological processes can be used to assess the disposition of single and multiple dose escalation studies, identify potentially saturable hepatic pathways, and assess the formation of metabolites. From this information, potential DDIs can be predicted and investigated.

In order to effectively utilize the drug metabolism and pharmacokinetic (DMPK) information generated from *in vitro* and *in vivo* studies, it is important to have a proper understanding of when in the development timeline the data should be generated. Additionally, a thorough understanding of the clearance mechanism of a chemical entity can help lessen the need for some downstream *in vivo* studies potentially saving the pharmaceutical organization hundreds of thousands of dollars. While the timing of specific investigations may change due to the nature of the chemical entity being tested, the following general DMPK chronology and endpoints should be considered during discovery and development [3, 4]. The bullets relating to drug metabolism are bolded for emphasis and will be expanded in greater detail in the following pages.

1. Lead Selection (Hit-to-Lead; 100s to 1000s of compounds across multiple chemical series)

   - Plasma protein binding, red blood cell partitioning, and intestinal permeability (Caco-2) assessments

   - ***In vitro* metabolic stability screening using hepatocytes, microsomes, and S9 fractions**

   - *In vivo* rodent PK studies

   - Investigate the *in vitro:in vivo* correlation (IVIVC) of CL and $t_{1/2}$ and identify the series with problematic kinetics (e.g., high CL or low $t_{1/2}$)

   - Identification of the relevant tissues where the chemical entity and metabolites may be sequestered

2. Optimization (Lead series identified and evaluated; <100 compounds)

   - Pharmacokinetic studies in rodent and nonrodent species

   - **Identification of clinically relevant DDIs (*In vitro* assessment of P450 induction and P450 inhibition)**

   - **Screening Cocktail DDI Study**

   - ***In vitro* soft spot analysis/metabolic identification to identify metabolically liable sites on investigated chemical entities**

   - **Drug transporter and tissue sequestration assessments**

   - Pharmacokinetic-Pharmacodynamic (PK-PD; exposure-effect) modeling

3. Drug Candidate Selection (< 5 compounds evaluated)

   - **Mass balance study in rodents and nonrodents in order to support nonrodent toxicology species selection**

- Allometric scaling to predict human $t_{1/2}$ and exposures in order to identify the starting dosages to be evaluated in the Phase 1 first-in-human (FIH) trials.

- **Evaluation of DDIs**

- **Metabolite profiling of high dose blood samples near the peak whole blood/plasma concentrations from the repeat-dose toxicity studies.**

4. Metabolite Safety Testing (Post FIH and concurrent with Phase 2 trials)

    - **Human specific metabolites or metabolites with exposures at higher levels in humans than in any of the animal test species are assessed in preclinical species.**

2. Lead selection

During the Lead Selection stage of drug discovery, candidate chemical series and potential lead compounds are screened for preferential physiochemical properties and metabolic stability. Promising chemical entities are then investigated *in vivo* in rodents (N = 3-5) via cassette dosing [5] in order to generate PK data. With recent advances in microsampling techniques [6] and automated blood sampling systems [7], robust PK data can be generated in a limited number of rodents resulting in reliable IVIVC models. Pharmacokinetic data can then be predicted across multiple species to evaluate and identify the chemical series and chemical entities that are ideal candidates for optimization.

Most chemical entities are substrates of *in vivo* enzymatic metabolic reactions that modify the chemical structure to clear the exogenous compound over time. Metabolizing enzymes are primarily expressed in the liver but are also found in the intestines, lungs, and other various organs. Traditionally, there are two phases of drug metabolism that exist to transfrom lipophilic compounds into hydrophilic products that are more readily eliminated from systemic circulation. Phase 1 biotransformations are primarily oxidative; however, reduction, hydrolysis, and hydration reactions are also observed. Phase 1 reactions are primarily carried out by microsomal expressed cytochrome P450s (CYP450), flavin monooxygenases, aldehyde oxidase, and monoamine oxidase in the hepatocytes and microsome preparations from hepatocytes (a fragment of endoplasmic reticulum and attached ribosomes obtained by the centrifugation of homogenized cells). Phase 2 biotransformations are conjugative and occur within the S9 fractions (harvested from a mixture of unfractionated microsomes and cytosol by the centrifugation [9000 g] of homogenized cells) and hepatocytes. The primary conjugative reactions are glucuronidation, sulfation, methylation, acetylation, glutathione conjugation, and amino acid conjugation.

2.1 Metabolic stability

The industry standard for screening the metabolic stability of a compound or compound-series is via the substrate depletion approach and the determination of half-life in rodent, nonrodent and human. Briefly, the metabolic stability, or intrinsic clearance (Cl_{int}) is assessed by incubating the compound at a concentration assumed to be below the K_m for P450 metabolism. The *in vitro* Cl_{int} can be assessed in multiple species hepatocytes, hepatic S9 fractions and/or microsomes [8]. A series of samples are collected and analyzed over the time course in order to determine the percentage of compound remaining. The resulting half-life ($t_{1/2}$) is then appropriately converted to an activity (Cl_{int}, mg/mL/Kg), taking into account the ratio of protein content to liver mass (e.g., mammalian microsomal protein, 45 mg protein/gm liver), and the ratio of liver mass to total animal or body mass (e.g., human, 20 gm/Kg body weight); the principles of allometry apply in this context of scaling protein content and P450 activity (physiological parameter) versus organ-to-body mass ratio (anatomical parameter) [9]. The intrinsic clearance *in vitro* PK parameter may be generated from a number of subcellular fractions, including microsomes, S9 fraction, cytosol and mitochondria (e.g., MAO metabolism), as well as from whole cell incubations employing freshly isolated or cryopreserved hepatocytes. The high throughput nature of the aforementioned metabolic stability assay enables the rapid generation of *in vitro* PK parameters ($t_{1/2}$ and Cl_{int}) with each cycle of medicinal chemistry. With the continued innovation of mass spectroscopy and the liquid chromatogram coupled mass spectrometry (LC/MS) bioanalytical techniques, the contemporary biotransformation laboratory and scientist can now identify metabolites in the same intrinsic clearance assay, thus elucidating the relevant pathway of metabolism under kinetically controlled conditions. Alternatively, the same subcellular fraction and whole cell metabolism experiment may be employed to determine all relevant pathways and under conditions where compound(s) concentrations have been elevated appreciably above the anticipated K_M for a particular drug metabolizing enzyme (DME). The merits of either approach will be discussed in a subsequent section.

2.2 Soft spot analysis/metabolite identification

The medicinal chemist utilizes the metabolic stability data generated during the Lead Selection and Lead Optimization stages of discovery as a tool to understand the impact of structural modifications within one or more chemical series or a lead series, respectively. Depending on the subcellular fraction employed, the Cl_{int} informs the chemist as to ensuing stabilization of the compound or series to oxidative (or reductive) metabolism via P450 (e.g., microsomes or S9 fractions). In addition to the $t_{1.2}$ and Cl_{int} data produced from *in vitro* screening, the incubations also provide an opportunity to determine the site of metabolism on the molecule, or elucidate the so-called metabolic "soft-spot". From P450 mediated oxidation, to direct glucuronidation and sulfation, to ester and amide hydrolysis, small molecule drug candidates possess physico-chemical properties that are perfectly suited to drug metabolism-mediated, hepatic clearance. Typically, the soft-spot analysis is performed in the same subcellular fraction or hepatocyte system employed in the intrinsic clearance assessment. With recent improvements in electrospray ionization liquid chromatography tandem mass spectrometry (ESI-LC–MS/MS) bioanalysis, the DMPK scientist is able to associate one or more predominate sites of metabolism (e.g., oxidation, reduction, hydrolysis, conjugation) with the clearance of a compound or series *in vitro*, and under the same kinetically controlled conditions of the metabolic stability assessment (i.e., $\leq 1\ \mu M$). The described soft-spot analysis construct enables a concerted execution of both the Cl_{int} assessment (substrate depletion) as well as the identification of the principal metabolites produced *in vitro* in "one plate". Whether in concert with the Cl_{int} assessment or as a discrete stand-alone in vitro experiment, innovation in mass spectroscopy hardware and software has enabled significant means of metabolite detection and structural elucidation, the results of which commonly augment the nonclinical pharmacology reports and summaries within an Investigational New Drug application (IND).

Still, the DMPK scientist may seize on the opportunity to determine the soft-spot(s) of metabolism to simultaneously assess the extent and range of biotransformation likely produced in multiple species during preclinical and clinical development. Access to study samples (e.g., plasma, urine, bile, feces, organ tissue) presents the opportunity to survey the metabolites produced in the rodent and nonrodent species selected for development, comparing to that observed in human hepatocytes and hepatic (e.g.) subcellular fractions. In order to provide a comparative analysis to the *in vivo* metabolism picture, the DMPK scientist will produce in parallel a set of *in vitro* experiments in rodent and nonrodent, where the compound or preclinical candidate is incubated at concentrations assumed to exceed the K_m for most drug metabolizing enzymes (e.g., ≥25 μM ≤50 μM). Importantly, *in vitro* incubations of subcellular fractions should be fortified with appropriate cofactors (or co-enzymes) to "fuel" the relevant catalytic activities of select enzymes and at excess (1-2 mM): P450 (NADPH, or NADPH-regenerating system), FMO (NADPH), UGT (UDPGA), SULT (PAPS), NAT (acetyl-CoA), GST (GSH).

2.3 *In vivo-in vitro* correlation

The *in vitro* hepatic clearance of a compound (within a series) is a valuable PK parameter for the medicinal chemist and the DMPK scientist. Because the intrinsic clearance (Cl_{int}, mL/min/kg) describes the unrestricted, unscaled clearance of a compound, the medicinal chemist may utilize Cl_{int} to gauge the impact of structural alterations in the series on P450 metabolism (oxidation or reduction in microsomes); the primary goal of which to stabilize a compound or chemical series towards hepatic clearance, thus increasing the *in vitro* half-life. The value of the Cl_{int} PK parameter is in its correlation to a plasma clearance (CL_p), as typically determined in a rodent (e.g., Sprague–Dawley rat) or nonrodent (e.g., beagle dog) species during the hit-to-lead and later in the lead optimization stages of discovery. Establishing an in *vitro:in vivo* correlation (IVIVC) between predicted hepatic clearance (CL_H) and CL_p serves two purposes: (1) validation of the CL_{int} screening approach for the ensuing lead optimization stage of discovery, and (2) establishes the nonclinical species for *in vivo* PK screening and the species predictive of human hepatic clearance. The selection of appropriate *in vitro* and *in vivo* PK screening approaches during early discovery provides a mechanism for an iterative medicinal chemistry optimization of one or more chemical series, with the goal of predicting human PK parameters.

3. Lead optimization

Once a lead series is selected, further *in vitro* and *in vivo* testing is conducted on a fewer number of compounds, illuminating metabolism and PK (and pharmacologic) attributes for select compounds. This stage of drug discovery is known as Lead Optimization. From an *in vitro* perspective, potential DDIs are identified with CYP450 inhibition and induction assays, and reaction phenotyping assays. Soft spot analysis is performed to identify areas liable to biotransformation, metabolic identification of potential *in vivo* metabolites, and drug transporters are identified for which the candidate entities are a substrate. Rodent and nonrodent PK studies are conducted in order to optimize the exposure and disposition (PK) of the lead series while determining the nonclinical pharmacologic effects of the lead series in select rodent and/or nonrodent disease models. These data are then used to establish preliminary exposure-effect relationships (PK-PD). The exposure data collected from rodent (e.g.) models of efficacy are particularly valuable and provide a critical assessment of dose-exposure relationships of the lead series in anticipation of advancing into the single- and repeat-dose tolerability assessments prior to candidate selection. At minimum this exposure information guides the discovery team to the dose range required for a tolerability screening assessment; ideally, the efficacy model exposure assessments guide the selection of the dosing frequency required to maintain exposure during the repeat-dose tolerability assessment.

The Food and Drug Administration's (FDA) January 2020 guidance on clinical drug interaction studies states that "clinically relevant DDIs between an investigational drug and other drugs should therefore be: (1) defined during drug development as part of the sponsor's assessment of the investigational drug's benefits and risks; (2) understood via nonclinical and clinical assessment at the time of the investigational drug's approval; (3) monitored after approval; and (4) communicated in the labeling." Furthermore, the FDA defines the goals of studies that evaluate P450 enzyme- and transporter-mediated DDIs to be: (1) determine whether the investigational drug alters the pharmacokinetics of other drugs; (2) determine whether other drugs alter the pharmacokinetics of the investigational drug; (3) determine the magnitude of changes in pharmacokinetic parameters; (4) determine the clinical significance of the observed or expected DDIs; and (5) inform the appropriate management and prevention strategies for clinically significant DDIs [10].

Additionally, the FDA also provided guidance for *in vitro* drug interaction studies (P450 and transporter) in January 2020. This guidance provides the framework for designing and conducting *in vitro* experiments in order to assess potential clinical DDIs. The CYP450 experiments are to: (1) determine which CYP450 enzyme the drug entity is a substrate of (reaction phenotyping); (2) determine if the drug entity is a CYP450 inhibitor; and (3) determine if the drug entity is a CYP450 inducer. Metabolite investigations may be warranted on a case-by-case basis. If the metabolite is pharmacologically active and contributes ≥50% of the overall activity, then reaction phenotyping analyses should be conducted. Inhibition studies are to be conducted if the total exposure/area under the curve (AUC) of the metabolite is ≥25% of the parent or if the metabolite is more polar than the parent entity and the AUC of the metabolite is greater than or equal to the parent. Transporter studies are to investigate if the drug entity is a substrate of efflux pumps (P-glycoprotein [P-gp] and breast cancer resistance protein [BCRP]), hepatic transporters (OATP1B1 and OATP1B3), and renal transporters (OAT, OCT, and MATE) [11].

3.1 Reaction phenotyping

Having assembled relative *in vitro* pharmacokinetic data (e.g., Cl_{int}) and elucidated metabolism pathways for a compound or preclinical candidate, it's incumbent upon the DMPK scientist to identify the particular human drug metabolizing enzymes that are contributing to the *in vitro* clearance in an effort to identify and/or manage latent drug–drug interaction potential that exist. To identify such victim drug–drug interaction (DDI) potential, [12] the DMPK scientist employs a variety of recombinantly expressed drug metabolizing enzymes, notably P450 enzymes to determine the extent any one enzyme contributes to the clearance of a compound [13]. The fraction-metabolized (f_m) term is often employed within the context of P450 mediated metabolism, but more recently applied to the growing number preclinical candidates observed to be non P450 substrates (e.g., UGT). Correlating the *in vitro* microsomal (e.g.) clearance to contributions from any one or more P450 enzymes, most notably P450 1A2, 2B6, 2C8, 2C9, 2C19, 2D6, and 3A4, is the goal of so-called reaction phenotyping. Importantly, this reaction phenotyping of drug clearance involves the comparative metabolism (and intrinsic clearance thereof) of the preclinical compound by the recombinant enzyme to what is observed in the subcelluar fraction; in the case of P450 or UGT, that can be accomplished in hepatic microsomes or S9 fractions. Two industrial standard approaches involve the generation of relative activity factors (RAF method) and intersystem extrapolation factors (ISEF) to adequately relate a single recombinant enzyme activity to human liver microsomes bearing a full complement of expressed P450 enzymes. Each of these methods, while instrumental in arriving at the f_m value for a particular drug candidate, fall short in estimating the impact of polymorphically expressed enzymes (e.g., P450 2D6, 2C9, 2C19, UGT1A1) in the metabolism-mediated clearance of a compound. More recently, and as a result of pharmacogenomics and pharmacogenetics clinical research and impact, the DMPK scientist can gain access to subcellular fractions obtained from sparse or densely genotyped individual liver donors.

The importance of linking a particular biotransformation reaction to one or more metabolites is of particular interest during preclinical development. Whether in terms of pharmacology (e.g., P450 mediated production of an active metabolite), drug safety (e.g., UGT mediated production of an acyl glucuronide) or confirming multiple enzymes producing the same pathway (e.g., risk mitigation of a clinically relevant DDI), the use of recombinantly expressed enzymes are critical in mapping the range of metabolites observed in human hepatocytes or subcellular fractions to specific drug metabolizing enzymes. At the elevated concentrations employed in the generation of metabolite(s) *in vitro*, there is limited kinetic value to these experiments and should be viewed as informative in nature and restricted to the metabolite ID and structure elucidation exercise previously described.

3.2 CYP450 inhibition studies

Once the metabolic pathways are identified, *in vitro* P450 inhibition and induction studies are conducted in order to predict clinically significant DDIs. Per the FDA's January 2020 guidance, "The sponsor should evaluate an investigational drug's potential to inhibit CYP1A2, CYP2B6, CYP2C8, CYP2C9, CYP2C19, CYP2D6, and CYP3A in both a reversible manner (i.e., reversible inhibition) and time-dependent manner (i.e., time-dependent inhibition (TDI))" [14].

In general, each microsomal assay includes the preparation of both test compound and positive control samples in order to assess the metabolite formation specific to each CYP450 isoform. Experiments are typically prepared with both the test compound at increasing concentrations and a selective P450 probe substrate prepared at a predetermined concentration that will produce first-order kinetics. Following an incubation under physiologic conditions (pH and temperature), the experiment is quenched and resulting incubations are prepared for analysis employing LC–MS/MS. The data is then analyzed by comparing the metabolite formation of the test samples relative to the control samples and dose–response plots are created to determine the specific endpoints of the assay.

3.3 Screening DDI cocktail assay

Concurrent with the early optimization stage P450 assessments, a cocktail of the test compound and substrates that exclusively bind to specific P450 isoforms is incubated with human liver microsomes across multiple concentrations of the test compound. Following incubation, P450 isoform specific metabolites are measured in each sample and compared to a control sample. Based on the metabolite abundance of the test samples relative to the control sample, as measured by liquid chromatography and tandem mass spectrometry (LC–MS/MS), a potential DDI liability can be identified early to inform future *in vitro* and potentially future *in vivo* investigations. Based on the results of this screening assay and the P450 inhibition and induction assays, definitive *in vitro* DDI screening may be warranted during the Drug Candidate Selection stage.

3.4 CYP450 induction studies

CYP induction is typically measured *in vitro* using three separate lots of human hepatocytes. A metabolically active human hepatocyte cell line (e.g. HepaRG) can sometimes be substituted for one of the human hepatocyte lots. Three P450s are commonly measured for induction – CYP1A2, 2B6 and 3A4. If CYP3A4 induction is observed, it is recommended to assess CYP2C8, 2C9 and 2C19 induction in a separate experiment. For the induction experiment, human hepatocytes are incubated in a sandwich culture format prior to the experiment. The media is changed to serum-free prior to the start of the experiment in order to lower the basal expression of CYPs. On day one, test compounds are added and incubated with the cells for 48-72 hours, with daily replenishment of media and test compound. Induction can be assessed by either measuring mRNA levels or activity levels. For the mRNA method, the cells are harvested after 48 hours, mRNA is extracted and the expression level of CYPs is measured by qPCR. For the activity assay, specific substrates for each of the CYPs are added following 72 hours of incubation and the rate of metabolism is measured over a defined time point, e.g. 2 hours. A positive result is considered to be ≥2-fold increase over the vehicle control.

3.5 Membrane drug transporters

Membrane drug transporters play an important role in the uptake, distribution and elimination of both endogenous substances and drugs in the body. Because they help regulate the flux of many substances across cell membranes they are often implicated in detoxification mechanisms, multidrug resistance and clinical DDIs [15]. Drug transporters control the concentration of drug substrates available for P450 reactions by regulating drug disposition within the cell for both the parent drug and metabolites. Drug metabolizing enzymes are often coupled with transporters to efficiently modify the level of drug present in a specific tissue. A well-known example of this is the efficient removal of bilirubin from plasma by OATP1B1-mediated uptake into the liver, UGT1A1-mediated formation of mono- and diglucuronide metabolites and subsequent elimination into the bile via the MRP2 transporter. In addition, the expression levels of drug metabolism enzymes are closely tied to transporters. For example, the nuclear receptor PXR regulates the expression of both drug metabolism enzymes such as CYP3A4 and CYP2C9 as well as several efflux drug transporters including P-gp and MRP2.

Membrane transporters relevant to drug development include two major superfamilies – ATB-binding cassette (ABC) and solute carrier (SLC). Members of the ABC superfamily utilize ATP hydrolysis to actively transport a solute across a cell membrane against a concentration gradient. The most relevant ABC transporters include P-glycoprotein (P-gp, MDR1), breast cancer resistance protein (BCRP) and multidrug resistance-associated protein 2 (MRP2). One of the primary functions of these transporters is to efflux small molecule substrates out of the cell in order to reduce cellular exposure and protect cells and organs against potentially harmful drugs or toxins. They are widely expressed in the epithelia of the intestine, liver and kidney, and in the endothelium of the blood–brain barrier and other blood-tissue barriers where they are localized on apical membranes.

In contrast, members of the SLC superfamily utilize solute exchange mechanisms to drive drug transport, including endogenous anions/cations or electrogenic mechanisms. SLC transporters include the major uptake transporters such as organic anion (OAT, OATP), organic cation (OCT) and the multidrug and toxin extrusion transporters (MATE1, MATE2-K). OATP1B1 and OATP1B3 are located primarily on the hepatocyte plasma-facing apical membrane, while OAT1, OAT3 and OCT2 are located on the basolateral membrane of the kidney proximal tubule. MATE1 and MATE2-K are located both in the proximal tubule and in the liver (canalicular membrane).

Several of the ATP and SLC transporters have been implicated in clinical DDIs and the FDA has focused on the following list as relevant for *in vitro* screening: P-gp, BCRP, OATP1B1, OATP1B3, OAT1, OAT3, OCT2, MATE1, and MATE2-K. *In vitro* evaluation of specific transporter interactions can employ a variety of tools including human and animal monolayer systems, transfected cell lines with single or multiple transporters over-expressed and membrane vesicles, along with a panel of substrates and inhibitors as control probes (**Table 1**).

3.5.1 Monolayer systems

The standard assay format for transporter function involves measuring the permeability of a test article through a confluent monolayer of cells grown on a permeable membrane. The cells and membrane are part of a transwell insert which fits into a normal 24-well plate, thus creating two media chambers. The upper reservoir is referred to as the apical (or A) chamber while the lower is the basolateral (or B) chamber. Addition of test article to each reservoir in separate wells, allows measurement of the apparent permeability in both directions (A to B, and B to A). The cell line used, therefore, must have the ability to form tight junctions between cells to prevent leakage of test article through the monolayer, and must express the transporters in a polarized fashion, enabling measurement of transport of substrates in two directions. Two cell lines are commonly used in this format – Caco-2 and MDCKII. The Transwell format is used not only to measure the permeability of the test article in a single direction, but also determine the efflux ratio, calculated as the ratio of permeability in both directions (B to A/A to B). If the efflux ratio is greater than 2, an interaction with a transporter is probable and needs further study.

Caco-2 cells were originally derived from a human colorectal adenocarcinoma. Although the cells originated from the human colon, they are widely used as a model of intestinal absorption and transporter activity [16]. When placed in culture, these cells undergo differentiation to an intestinal phenotype. The cells are characterized by a well-defined apical brush border, formation of tight junctions, and the endogenous expression of the majority of uptake and efflux transporters normally present in intestinal enterocytes [17]. Caco-2 cells are regarded as the most sophisticated *in vitro* tool for medium to high throughput modeling of drug transport across human plasma/tissue barriers.

A non-human alternative cell line that is also widely used in monolayer studies is MDCKII (Madin-Darby canine kidney strain II). A number of MDCKII cell lines

Assay	Cell system	Endpoint
Permeability Assessment	Caco-2, MDCK	Apparent permeability (P_{app}), efflux ratio
ATP Transporters (efflux)	Caco-2, MDCK, membrane vesicles, genetically modified cell lines	Substrate/Inhibitor
SLC Transporters (uptake)	Hepatocytes, transfected cells (MDCK, HEK293, CHO)	Substrate/Inhibitor

Table 1.
Examples of in vitro *systems to investigate transporter-mediated drug interactions.*

have been generated with single or double human transporters transfected into the cells. These modified animal cell lines enable the study of individual human transporters in the absence of competition from other human transporters. One caveat with MDCK cells is that there is an active form of canine P-gp present that is functionally similar to the human form and needs to be accounted for when transporter data is analyzed.

Other animal cell lines used for transporter studies include LLC-PK1 (porcine) and Chinese hamster ovary (CHO) cells.

3.5.2 Membrane vesicle assays

An alternative to cell-based transporter assays involves membrane vesicles, in which the assay is conducted with membrane preparations from baculovirus-infected insect cells or mammalian cells that have been transfected with the transporter of interest. When isolated, a small portion of the membrane vesicles end up in an inverted configuration ("inside-out") and are particularly useful for studying efflux transporters. Transporter activity (activation or inhibition) can be assessed by either measuring uptake of a substrate into the vesicles over time, or by measuring ATPase activity.

3.5.3 Genetically modified cell lines

Transporters recognize and interact with of a broad range of compounds, and each transporter has been characterized for their physicochemical preferences in substrates [18]; however, there remains a large overlapping area of substrate recognition between transporters. Some of the current ambiguity in assigning specificity toward a single transporter is due to the use of different cellular systems to define the interaction. Small molecule inhibitors are commonly used to define transporter interactions, but inhibitors often show overlapping interactions between transporters [19]. Novel test systems that avoid the use of small molecule inhibitors may be able to improve our ability to unambiguously identify specific substrate interactions Two approaches have recently been used to address this situation. Knockdown of transporter gene expression can be accomplished using small inhibitory RNA (siRNA). Alternatively, complete gene knockout can be accomplished using zinc finger nucleases (ZFNs) or Clustered Regularly Interspaced Short Palindromic Repeats (CRISPR). For example, several individual or dual knockout cell lines were recently developed in the C2BBe1 cell line (a subclone of Caco-2) and are commercially available [20]. In addition, the canine P-gp transporter in MDCK cells has recently been knocked out.

4. Drug candidate selection

Following the investigations of the Lead Optimization stage, the pharmaceutical organization should have weaned their list of promising drug candidates to less than five entities. From a drug metabolism perspective, there are three major investigations that occur: (1) ADME profiling in rodents and nonrodent species; (2) definitive *in vitro* DDI screening and potentially *in vivo* confirmatory investigations; and (3) metabolite profiling in the identified toxicology species. By the end of the Drug Candidate Selection stage, the pharmaceutical organization should have all the information they need to support their Investigational New Drug application (IND) or Exploratory IND application.

4.1 Mass balance study

Due to the high expense, complete ADME profiling (non-radiolabeled) does not typically occur until a strong candidate for IND submission has been identified. The *in vitro* metabolism, tissue distribution analyses, and *in vivo* PK studies performed in the prior development stages are used to inform the investigators regarding the potential route of clearance, the tissues to be collected and quantitated, and if a major metabolite should be investigated as part of the study. The goals of these studies are to definitively identify the route of elimination (including biliary excretion), assess tissue distribution, and if applicable, characterize metabolite exposure relative to parent exposures. The animals in these studies are typically split into two groups where one group has their bile duct cannulated in order to assess biliary excretion from the liver. The animals are individually housed in metabolism cages that collect the urine and feces excreted by each animal. Depending on the study design, each animal may be sacrificed at various time points in order to assess critical tissues for exposure to the drug entity.

4.2 DDI evaluation

Based on the results of the P450 inhibition/induction assays and the screening DDI studies, specific P450 isoforms are further investigated *in vitro* for the DDI potential instead of a general cocktail approach as employed in the Lead Optimization stage. If an *in vitro* DDI is observed, an *in vivo* study is warranted to confirm if the DDI persists.

4.3 Metabolite profiling

At dose levels greater than 100 mg/kg, the primary clearance mechanism is typically saturated resulting in greater interaction between the drug entity and other P450 enzymes. Metabolite profiling analyses typically use blood samples collected at tox level doses greater than 100 mg/kg; ideally samples at or near the C_{max}. The metabolites are typically identified early during the lead optimization stage in the soft spot/metabolite identification studies. The parent and metabolites are typically quantitated via LC–MS/MS methods. The end goal is to obtain the percent abundance of each metabolite relative to the parent.

5. Metabolite safety testing

Following Phase 1 FIH studies, the blood samples at or near the C_{max} from the high dose cohort of the multiple ascending dose study undergo metabolite profiling. The resulting metabolite abundancies are then compared to the preclinical metabolite profiling studies in order to identify human only metabolites or metabolites that are present at higher plasma concentrations in humans than in the animals used in the preclinical studies. These metabolites are referred to as disproportionate drug metabolites. Per the FDA's March 2020 guidance, "In general, these metabolites are of interest if they account for plasma levels greater than 10 percent of total drug-related exposure, measured as area under the curve at steady state." In the instance that a disproportionate meets these criteria, futher *in vitro* (genotoxicity) and *in vivo* (general toxicity and embryo-fetal development toxicity) studies are required to assess the safety of the metabolite. Typically, these studies can be conducted concurrently with Phase 2 studies prior to the large-scale Phase 3 trials.

6. Summary

Drug metabolism is a drug-clearing event from systemic circulation influencing efficacy and toxicity in humans and preclinical species. The primary endpoints of enzymatic metabolism studies in both the drug discovery and preclinical stages are to resolve metabolic stability, identify and quantify primary metabolites, identify metabolic routes, and measure the potential for DDIs and are used to predict human PK. The intrinsic kinetic properties of the chemical entity with consideration of the physiological processes can be used to assess the disposition of single and multiple dose escalation studies, identify potentially saturable hepatic and transporter pathways, and assess the formation of metabolites. From this information, potential DDIs are predicted and subsequently investigated.

Author details

Benjamin Mann*, Roger Melton and David Thompson
Inotiv, St. Louis, Missouri, United States of America

*Address all correspondence to: bmann@inotivco.com

References

[1] Pelkonen O, Turpeinen M, Uusitalo J, Rautio A, Raunio H. Prediction of drug metabolism and interactions on the basis of in vitro investigations. Basic Clin Pharmacol Toxicol. 2005; 96(3):167-175. DOI: 10.1111/j.1742-7843.2005.pto960305.x

[2] Balani SK, Miwa GT, Gan LS, Wu JT, Lee FW. Strategy of utilizing in vitro and in vivo ADME tools for lead optimization and drug candidate selection. Curr Top Med Chem. 2005;5(11):1033-8. DOI: 10.2174/156802605774297038

[3] Zhang D, Luo G, Ding X, Lu C. Preclinical experimental models of drug metabolism and disposition in drug discovery and development. Acta Pharmaceutica Sinica B, 2012:2(6). DOI: 10.1016/j.apsb.2012.10.004

[4] Balani SK, Miwa GT, Gan LS, Wu JT, Lee FW. Strategy of utilizing in vitro and in vivo ADME tools for lead optimization and drug candidate selection. Curr Top Med Chem. 2005;5(11):1033-8. DOI: 10.2174/156802605774297038

[5] Bridges TM, Morrison RD, Byers FW, Luo S, Scott Daniels J. Use of a novel rapid and resource-efficient cassette dosing approach to determine the pharmacokinetics and CNS distribution of small molecule 7-transmembrane receptor allosteric modulators in rat. Pharmacol Res Perspect. 2014;2(6): e00077. DOI: 10.1002/prp2.77

[6] Bridges TM, Morrison RD, Byers FW, Luo S, Scott Daniels J. Use of a novel rapid and resource-efficient cassette dosing approach to determine the pharmacokinetics and CNS distribution of small molecule 7-transmembrane receptor allosteric modulators in rat. Pharmacol Res Perspect. 2014;2(6): e00077. DOI: 10.1002/prp2.77

[7] Kamendi HW, Brott DA, Chen Y, Litwin DC, Lengel DJ, Fonck C, Bui KH, Gorko MA, Bialecki RA. Combining radio telemetry and automated blood sampling: A novel approach for integrative pharmacology and toxicology studies. Journal of Pharmacological and Toxicological Methods. 2010;62(1):30-9. DOI: 10.1016/j.vascn.2010.01.014

[8] Obach RS, Reed-Hagen AE. Measurement of Michaelis constants for cytochrome P450-mediated biotransformation reactions using a substrate depletion approach. Drug Metab Dispos. 2002;30(7):831-7. DOI: 10.1124/dmd.30.7.831

[9] Obach RS, Baxter JG, Liston TE, Silber BM, Jones BC, MacIntyre F, Rance DJ, Wastall P. The prediction of human pharmacokinetic parameters from preclinical and in vitro metabolism data. J Pharmacol Exp Ther. 1997;283(1): 45-58.

[10] U.S. Department of Health and Human Services Food and Drug Administration Center for Drug Evaluation and Research (CDER). Clinical Drug Interaction Studies— Cytochrome P450 Enzyme- and Transporter-Mediated Drug Interactions [Internet]. 2020. Available from: https://www.fda.gov/regulatory-information/search-fda-guidance-documents/clinical-drug-interaction-studies-cytochrome-p450-enzyme-and-transporter-mediated-drug-interactions

[11] U.S. Department of Health and Human Services Food and Drug Administration Center for Drug Evaluation and Research (CDER). In Vitro Drug Interaction Studies — Cytochrome P450 Enzyme- and Transporter-Mediated Drug Interactions [Internet]. 2020. Available from: https://www.fda.gov/regulatory-information/search-fda-guidance-documents/vitro-drug-interaction-studies-cytochrome-p450-enzyme-and-transporter-mediated-drug-interactions

[12] U.S. Department of Health and Human Services Food and Drug Administration Center for Drug Evaluation and Research (CDER). In Vitro Drug Interaction Studies — Cytochrome P450 Enzyme- and Transporter-Mediated Drug Interactions [Internet]. 2020. Available from: https://www.fda.gov/regulatory-information/search-fda-guidance-documents/vitro-drug-interaction-studies-cytochrome-p450-enzyme-and-transporter-mediated-drug-interactions

[13] Stringer RA, Strain-Damerell C, Nicklin P, Houston JB. Evaluation of recombinant cytochrome P450 enzymes as an in vitro system for metabolic clearance predictions. Drug Metab Dispos. 2009;37(5):1025-34. DOI: 10.1124/dmd.108.024810

[14] U.S. Department of Health and Human Services Food and Drug Administration Center for Drug Evaluation and Research (CDER). In Vitro Drug Interaction Studies — Cytochrome P450 Enzyme- and Transporter-Mediated Drug Interactions [Internet]. 2020. Available from: https://www.fda.gov/regulatory-information/search-fda-guidance-documents/vitro-drug-interaction-studies-cytochrome-p450-enzyme-and-transporter-mediated-drug-interactions

[15] International Transporter Consortium, Giacomini KM, et al. Membrane transporters in drug development. Nat Rev Drug Discov. 2010;9(3):215-36. DOI: 10.1038/nrd3028

[16] Van Breemen RB, Li Y. Caco-2 cell permeability assays to measure drug absorption. Expert Opin Drug Metab Toxicol. 2005;1(2):175-85. DOI: 10.1517/17425255.1.2.175

[17] Hilgendorf C, Ahlin G, Seithel A, Artursson P, Ungell AL, Karlsson J. Expression of thirty-six drug transporter genes in human intestine, liver, kidney, and organotypic cell lines. Drug Metab Dispos. 2007;35(8):1333-40. DOI: 10.1124/dmd.107.014902

[18] Lin X, Skolnik S, Chen X, Wang J. Attenuation of intestinal absorption by major efflux transporters: quantitative tools and strategies using a Caco-2 model. Drug Metab Dispos. 2011; 39(2):265-74. DOI: 10.1124/dmd.110.034629

[19] Matsson P, Pedersen JM, Norinder U, Bergström CA, Artursson P. Identification of novel specific and general inhibitors of the three major human ATP-binding cassette transporters P-gp, BCRP and MRP2 among registered drugs. Pharm Res. 2009;26(8):1816-31. DOI: 10.1007/s11095-009-9896-0

[20] Sampson KE, Brinker A, Pratt J, Venkatraman N, Xiao Y, Blasberg J, Steiner T, Bourner M, Thompson DC. Zinc finger nuclease-mediated gene knockout results in loss of transport activity for P-glycoprotein, BCRP, and MRP2 in Caco-2 cells. Drug Metab Dispos. 2015;43(2):199-207. DOI: 10.1124/dmd.114.057216

Section 2

Perspectives in Drug Metabolism

Chapter 3

From Pharmacogenetics to Gene Expression: Implications for Precision Medicine in Diabetes

Katy Sánchez-Pozos, María de los Ángeles Granados-Silvestre and María Guadalupe Ortíz-López

Abstract

Approximately 25–60% of patients show specific pharmacological responses to a particular drug. We call this interindividual variability (IV) response to drugs affecting their efficacy and the appearance of side effects in individuals. This IV may be due to multifactorial components such as genetic factors (single nucleotide polymorphisms, SNPs; and copy number variations, CNV), environmental stimuli, epigenetic modulation, disease/health conditions, or drug interactions, among others. Therefore, these factors can influence the response to the drug by modifying absorption, metabolism, pharmacokinetics (PK), and pharmacodynamics (PD), causing the loss of treatment efficacy or leading to adverse drug reactions with negative consequences for patients. The knowledge in pharmacogenetics (study of pharmacological consequences of single gene mutations) and pharmacogenomics (study of the influence of many gene or gene patterns in the reponse to drugs), disciplines that seek to predict how a specific individual responds to the administration of a particular drug, has advanced by leaps and bounds thanks to "omics" technologies. Nonetheless, despite, the development of next-generation sequencing platforms and the mapping of the human genome have transformed the field of pharmacogenetics, the translational into clinical practice has been slow. Therefore, identification of SNPs that could affect the expression of pharmacogenes in order to make associations with PK and PD will improve our understanding of genetic effects on drug efficacy and transfer it to the clinic. Type 2 diabetes (T2D) represents a national public health problem, not only because of the high frequency of the disease reported worldwide, but also because of the poor adherence to therapeutic management, whose causes have not yet been clarified. One of the challenges in the management of diseases to reach optimal treatment is the complex genetic background. Hence, the integration of multiple levels of pharmacological information, including variation in gene sequence, impact in drug response, and function of drug targets, could help us to predict sources of interpatient variability in drug effects, laying the basis for precision therapy. Thus, the present chapter aims to collect all the available data about genetic variations in pharmacogenes affecting drug response in T2D and integrate it with their effect on gene expression to elucidate their impact in pharmacological efficacy.

Keywords: diabetes, pharmacogenetics, pharmacogenes, expression

IntechOpen

1. Introduction

Although there is no consensus in the contribution of genetic component to drug response, many studies from the 1970s have estimated that could be between 20 and 95% of the variability in drug disposition and effects [1]. The difficulty in reaching a consensus is because the contribution of environmental and genetic components to pharmacogenetics cannot be evaluated, through only one approach, that is, analyzing only one drug or group of drugs, or only a SNP or a group of SNPs; we have to talk about PK, PD and related outcomes. In this context, there are a variety of studies focused on PK, or PD, but the convergence of all these concepts has been difficult, so the translation to the clinical practice has been challenging. Along with these barriers are additional factors, such as gene–environment interactions and gene–gene interactions [2]. Moreover, the different responses among ethnicities are another factor to add to this complex phenomenon.

The knowledge on which the participation of genetics in response to the action of drugs in an individual or group of individuals has been generated through various studies, applying different strategies such as those described below. In this regard, in past decades, different laboratories in four countries carried out twin studies with different drugs to determine the contribution of genetic and environmental factors to interindividual variations. The results from all studies converged in that PK variation were similar between monozygotic twins and was preserved within dizygotic twins, and even as similar as the monozygotic twins [3]. Researchers from these laboratories conclude that genetic factors primarily controlled interindividual variations in the metabolism of a wide range of drugs [3–8]. In the field of heritability of antidiabetics drug response, the studies are scarce, but one classic example is tolbutamide. In this context, an intravenous administration to 42 nondiabetic subjects, eight of their relatives, and to five sets of twins, the authors observed a monogenic control of tolbutamide revealed by a heritability value of 0.995 (this value means that considering a trait with 1.0 heritability, such as a Mendelian trait, the genetic factors have a great or complete influence in phenotype; in contrast, a trait with 0.0 heritability will not be influenced by genetic factors) [9]. In a more recent study by Gjesing et al., they found high heritabilities estimations for acute insulin secretion subsequent to glucose stimulation (0.88 ± 0.14), for insulin sensitivity (0.26 ± 0.12), disposition index (0.56 ± 0.14) and disposition index after tolbutamide administration (0.49 ± 0.14) in 284 non diabetic family members of patients with T2D after an intravenous injection of tolbutamide [10]. In another study of genome-wide complex trait analysis in patients in the Genetics of Diabetes Audit and Research in Tayside Scotland (GoDARTS) study, the heritability of glycaemic response to metformin varied by response phenotype, with a heritability of 34% ($p = 0{\cdot}022$) for the absolute reduction in HbA_{1c} in 2085 individuals in treatment with metformin [11]. Hence, these studies clearly show that the response to different types or classes of drugs is modulated by the individual's genetics and can be passed on to their descendants showing a clearly genetic component.

2. Variability in drug response in T2D

Diabetes has become a health problem (by 2030, the number of individuals with diabetes is estimated to rise to 578 million and 700 million by 2045) [12]. Approximately, 90–95% of cases of diabetes correspond to T2D. T2D is a chronic metabolic disease characterized by hyperglycemia, resulting from insulin resistance and reduced insulin secretion, which leads to impaired glucose utilization, dyslipidemia and hyperinsulinemia [13].

The great prevalence of T2D impacts both direct and indirect costs. In 2019, the International Diabetes Federation estimated that total diabetes-related health spending reached $ 760 billion. By the years 2030 and 2045, spending is forecast to reach $ 825 billion and $ 845 billion, respectively [12]. Moreover, approximately the 32% of annual costs per diabetic patient is destined to treatment [14]. Furthermore, approximately 50% of T2D patients have good glycemic control considering HbA1c < 7%, which means that ~50% have poor glycemic control [15]. Besides, as consequence of adverse drug reactions (approximately 20–30%) there is a high prevalence of treatment abandonment [16–18] All these facts denote the need for new drugs or strategies to improve glycemic control. Current treatment to control diabetes is aimed at specific key targets in glucose metabolism such as: adipose and muscle tissue to reduce insulin resistance, or act on the liver to inhibit glucose production, as well as stimulate the pancreas to release insulin. However, it is necessary to go beyond lowering glucose levels. In clinical practice it is often observed that T2D patients who receive identical antidiabetic regimens have significant variability in drug response, hence interindividual variation may be caused by numerous factors, such as genetic factors, physical inactivity, hypertension, age, gender and others [19]. Particularly, the genetic variability of therapy response was recently shown in several independent studies for the common drugs used for T2D treatment. Therefore, identification of genetic variants and their impact in drug response may improve our knowledge in the field, in order to be able of translate it into clinical practice. This could help in decision making on the therapeutic approach, reducing the rates of side effects and improving the adherence to treatment. Thus, the present chapter aims to collect all the available data about genetic variations in pharmacogenes affecting drug response in T2D and integrate them with their effect on gene expression, and to elucidate their impact on pharmacological efficacy.

In order to cover the objective, we compile all the available information about pharmacogenetics and epigenetics in T2D. We carried out a literature search using PubMed and Google Scholar. For this purpose, search words used were the following: diabetes + pharmacogenetics (826 studies); type 2 diabetes + pharmacogenetics (421 studies), diabetes + pharmacogenomics (1,184 studies); type 2 diabetes + pharmacogenomics (456 studies). When we added the words "drug response" the result was 338 and 267 papers, for pharmacogenomics and pharmacogenetics, respectively; or when we added the words "personalized medicine" in the search, we retrieved 152 and 114 papers, for pharmacogenomics and pharmacogenetics, respectively. **Table 1** shows all the studies considered significantly associated with antidiabetics drug response. Regarding the Epigenetics section, this was covered with a literature search using the words diabetes + drug response + epigenetics. **Table 2** shows the reports of epigenetics variations that influence drug response in T2D treatment. All the studies were chosen taking into account glycemic control and significance.

2.1 Single nucleotide polymorphisms

SNPs, are modifications in the DNA sequence, that implies changes in single nucleotides, which are the most common variations and the main source of interindividual diversity [99]. Interindividual variability could be explained in part by SNPs in genes encoding drug-metabolizing enzymes, transporters, receptors and molecules involved in drug metabolism. In this context, many SNPs related with the metabolism of antidiabetic drugs have been described. In the following section we

Drug group	Gene (Encoded protein)	dbSNP ID	Aminoacid change	Population	Effect	References
Biguanides (Metformin)	*SLC22A1* (OCT1)	rs12208357	Arg61Cys	European	Association with metformin intolerance	[20–22]
		rs72552763	Met420del			
		rs34059508	Gly465Arg			
		rs34130495	Gly401Ser		Lower decrease in HbA1c	
		rs1867351	Ser52Ser	Asian	Reductions in PPG and ΔHbA1c	[23]
		rs622342	Intron A > C	South Indian	Less response to metformin	[24]
				European	Decreased reduction in HbA1c levels	[25]
				Mexican	High ΔHbA1c values	[26]
		rs36056065	Indel GTAAGTTG	European	Association with metformin side effects	[27]
		rs628031	Val408Met	Mexican	High ΔHbA1c values	[26]
				Chinese	Reduction in ΔHbA1c and ΔFPG	[23]
				European	Association with metformin side effects	[27]
		rs594709	597 A > G	Mexican	Increase in HbA1c values	[26]
				Chinese	Increase in FINS decrease in HOMA-IS and in QUICKI	[28]
		rs145450955	Thr201Met	Iranian	High HbA1c values	[29]
	SLC22A2 (OCT2)	rs316019	Ala270Ser	Chinese	Higher incidence of hyperlactacidemia	[30–32]
				South Indian	Better response	
		rs3119309	Intergenic	European	Association with metformin inefficiency	[33]
		rs7757336				
		rs2481030				

Drug group	Gene (Encoded protein)	dbSNP ID	Aminoacid change	Population	Effect	References
	SLC47A1 (MATE1)	rs2252281	g. − 66 T → C	European African American	Enhanced response	[34]
		rs2289669	g. − 130G → A	European	Association with reduction in HbA1c levels	[35]
	SLC47A2 (MATE2)	rs12943590	Gly211Val		Reduced response	[34]
				South Indian	Better response	[31]
		rs34399035	Gly393Arg	European	Lower decrease in HbA1c	[22]
	SLC2A2 (GLUT2)	rs8192675	Intron C > T	European American African American Asian American Latino	Reduction in HbA1c values	[36, 37]
					Reduction in blood glucose	
	C11orf65 (MFI)	rs11212617	Intron C > A	European	Association with treatment success	[38]
	CPA6 (CBPA6)	rs2162145	UTR variant T > A / C/G	European African American	Better response	[39]
	PRPF31 (PRP31)	rs254271	Intron T > A /C/G		Worse response	
	STK11	rs2075604	Intron G > T	Chinese	Better therapeutic efficacy	[32]
	CAPN10 (CAN10)	rs3792269	Arg197Gly	European African American	Association with less treatment success and with smaller reduction in HbA1c	[40]
	SP1	rs784892	Intron G > A	European American African American Asian American	Association with decreased efficacy	[41]

Drug group	Gene (Encoded protein)	dbSNP ID	Aminoacid change	Population	Effect	References
	FMO5	rs7541245	Intron C > A	Not provided	Association with decreased glycemic response (decrease response to metformin)	[42]
	SLC22A3 (OCT3)	rs2076828	C > G	European African American	Association with reduced response	[43]
Sulfonylureas	*CYP2C9*	rs1799853 (*2)	Arg144Cys	European	Greater response to sulfonylureas	[44, 45]
		rs1057910 (*3)	Ile359Leu	Mexican	Association with good glycemic control	
	ABCC8	rs757110	Ser1369Ala	Chinese	Association with FPG, 2 h plasma glucose and HbA1c decrease	[46, 47]
					Association with therapeutic efficacy	
		rs1799854	Intron C > T	European	Lower HbA1c concentration	[48]
		rs1799859	Arg1273Arg			
		rs1801261	Thr759Thr	Chinese	Less reduction in FPG and HbA1c levels	[49]
	KCNJ11 (KCJ11)	rs5219	Glu23Lys	European Chinese	Better response	[50, 51]
				Mexican	Lower response	[52]
		rs5210	UTR G > A	Chinese	Association with FPG decrease	[46]
	KCNQ1	rs163184	C > G	European	Lower FPG response	[53]
		rs2237892	Intron C > T	Chinese	Association with treatment success	[54]
		rs2237895	Intron A > C, T		Association with treatment success	
	TCF7L2 (TF7L2)	rs7903146	Intron C > T	European	Lower effect of gliclazide	[55]
		rs12255372	Intron G > T		Association with therapeutic failure	[56, 57]
	NOS1AP (CAPON)	rs10494366	Intron G > C/T		Less effectiveness of treatment	[58]

Drug group	Gene (Encoded protein)	dbSNP ID	Aminoacid change	Population	Effect	References
	IRS1	rs1801278	Gly972Arg	African	Association with increased risk for secondary failure	[59, 60]
				European		
	ABCA1	rs9282541	Arg230Cys	Mexican	Association with decreased response to treatment	[61]
Thiazolidinediones	*PPARG2* (PPARγ2)	rs1801282	Pro12Ala	Chinese	Association with better response	[62, 63]
					Higher ΔFPG	
		rs880663	Intron A > G	Mexican American	Association with response to troglitazone	[64]
		rs4135263	Intron T > C			
		rs1152003	G > C			
		rs6806708	G > T			
		rs13065455	C > A/G			
		rs13088205	T > G			
		rs13088214	T > C			
		rs13073869	Intron G > A/C			
	PPARGC1A (PGC-1α)	rs8192678	Gly482Ser	Chinese	Reduced ΔFPG and ΔFINS	[65]
		rs2970847	Thr394Thr		Reduced ΔPINS	
	UCP2	rs659366	−866 G/A	Chinese	Smaller attenuated PINS and greater attenuated HbA1c	[66]
	CYP2C8	rs10509681 (*3)	Lys399Arg	European	Association with reduced glycemic response	[67]
	SLCO1B1	rs4149056	Val174Ala	European	Association with enhanced glycemic response	[67]

Drug group	Gene (Encoded protein)	dbSNP ID	Aminoacid change	Population	Effect	References
	KCNQ1	rs2237892	Intron C > T	Chinese	Larger augmentation in Δ2h glucose	[54]
		rs2237895	Intron A > C/T		Greater decrement in ΔHbA1c	
	ADIPOQ (ADPN)	rs266729	−11377 C > G		Attenuated rosiglitazone effect	[68]
		rs2241766	GLy15Gly		Attenuated ΔFINS	
					Greater decrease in HbA1c and association with pioglitazone treatment	[69]
		rs1501299	SNP + 276 G > T	Korean	Smaller reductions in FPG and HbA1c	[70]
		rs182052	−10068 G > A	Chinese	Increased reduction in HbA1c	[71]
	RETN	rs1862513	−420 C > G	Japanese	Correlation with reduction of HbA1c	[72]
	LEP	rs7799039	G-2548A	Chinese	High differential values of FINS and PINS	[73]
	TNFA	rs1800629	G-308A		Lower values of FINS	
	PTPRD	rs17584499	Intron C > T		Higher ΔPPG	[63]
DPP-4 inhibitors	*TCF7L2* (TF7L2)	rs7903146	Intron C > T	European African Asian	Lower reduction of HbA1c	[74]
	KCNJ11 (KCJ11)	rs2285676	UTR A > G/T	Asian	Association with better response	[75]
	CTRB1/2	rs7202877	T > C/G	European	Smaller decrease of HbA1c	[76]
	KCNQ1	rs163184	Intron T > C/G		Association with a reduced glycemic response	[77]
	GLP1R	rs3765467	Arg131Gln	Korean	Association with HbA1c reduction	[78–80]
		rs6923761	Gly168Ser	European		
	DPP4	rs2909451	Intron C > T	Not Provided	Association with DPP-4 activity	[81]
		rs759717	Intron G > C			
		rs6733162	Intron G > C/A			

DOI: http://dx.doi.org/10.5772/intechopen.97375

Drug group	Gene (Encoded protein)	dbSNP ID	Aminoacid change	Population	Effect	References
	PRKD1	rs57803087	Intron A > G	Taiwanese	Association with DPP-4 inhibitor response	[82]
	ABCB1 (MDR1)	rs1128503	Gly412Gly	Asian	Association with response to therapy	[83]
	CDKAL1	rs7754840	Intron C > G	Japanese	Association with HbA1c reduction	[84]
		rs7756992	Intron A > G			
GLP-1 receptor agonists	GLP1R	rs10305420	Pro7Leu	Chinese		[85]
	TCF7L2 (TF7L2)	rs7903146	Intron C > T	Brazilian	Association with PINS	[86]
		rs761386	Intron C > G/T	Taiwanese	Association with changes in the standard deviation of plasma glucose	[87]
	SORCS1 (SORC1)	rs1416406	A > G/T	Chinese	Association with FINS	[88]
	CNR1	rs1049353	Thr453Thr	European	Association with improvement of insulin resistance	[89]
SGLT2 inhibitors	*UGT1A9*	rs72551330	Met33Thr	Not Provided	Higher AUC (26%)	[90, 91]
	SLC5A2 (SGLT2)	rs9934336	Intron G > A	European	Association with reduced 30-min plasma glucose	[92]

OR: Odd ratio; BG: Blood glucose; FINS: Fasting serum insulin; PINS: Postprandial serum insulin; PPG: Postprandial plasma glucose; HOMA-IS: Insulin sensitivity by homeostasis model assessment; HOMA-IR: Insulin resistance by homeostasis model assessment; HOMA-BCF: homeostatic index of percentage of β-cell function; FBG: fasting blood glucose; FG: fasting glucose; AUC: Area under the curve. The gray cells indicate a haplotype associated with metformin intolerance in the study of Dujic et al. in 2015 [21].

Table 1.
Changes in DNA sequence that influence T2D treatment.

Drug group	Gene /miRNA (Encoded protein)	CpG site	Effect	References
Biguanides (Metformin)	CFAP58 (CFA58)	cg03529510	Association with glycemic metformin response	[93]
	OR4S1	cg05402062		
	GPHA2	cg16704073		
	SAP130 (SP130)	cg16240962		
	SEPT11 (SEP11)	cg01070242		
	LRRN2	cg05151280		
	CSTT	cg07511259		
	SCYL1	cg27553780	Association with metformin intolerance	
	FOXA2 (HNF-3B)	cg12356107		
	PGM1	cg02994863		
	FAM107A (F107A)	cg08148545		
	SLC22A1 (OCT1)	cg24864413	Lower DNA methylation and lower glucose levels	[94]
	SLC22A3 (S22A3)	cg06295784		
		cg07883823		
	SLC47A1 (MATE1)	cg01530032		
		cg07829432		
		cg12550399		
	miR-192	N. A.	Decreased fasting glucose and HbA1c	[95, 96]
	miR-140-5p			
	miR-222			
Sulfonyulureas	KCNJ11 (KCJ11)	N.R..	26.2% vs. 27.2%	[97]
	ABCC8		0% vs. 7.2%	
SGLT2 inhibitors	miR30e-5p	N. A.	Upregulated	[98]
	miR199a3p		Downregulated	

N.R. Not reported.

Table 2.
Epigenetics variations that influence T2D treatment.

described the most significant SNPs associated with drug response, specifically glycemic control, with antidiabetics treatment.

2.1.1 Biguanides (Metformin)

First-line drugs in T2D therapy are biguanides, however, when the patient is not obese, the sulfonylureas group is usually prescribed and the response to treatment will be evaluated after 3 months [100]. Guidelines from the American Diabetes Association/European Association for the Study of Diabetes (ADA/EASD) and the American Association of Clinical Endocrinologists/American College of Endocrinology (AACE/ACE) recommend early initiation of metformin as a first-line drug for monotherapy and combination therapy for patients with T2D [101]. Approximately 30% of patients with T2D do not respond to metformin and about 20 to 30% experience intolerable side effects [102]. There is considerable variability in the glycemic response and PK characteristics of metformin. In terms of PK, metformin is not metabolized, and is excreted unchanged in the urine, with a half-life of roughly 5 h. In particular, mean plasma concentrations of metformin fluctuate between 0.4 and 1.3 mg/L at a dose of 1,000 mg twice daily [103].

The disposition of metformin includes elimination and tissue distribution, which in turn involves organic transporters (OCTs) and multidrug and toxin extrusion proteins (MATEs); both may contribute to the wide variation in metformin PK. Metformin response variability is important, in fact >30% of patients receiving metformin are classified as poor responders [102]. This drug is a polar molecule largely eliminated by the kidney without undergoing hepatic metabolization. The processes of uptake and secretion of metformin are highly dependent on membrane transporters, among which are solute carrier family 22A members 1 and 2 (SLC22A1/OCT1 and SLC22A2/OCT2, respectively), multidrug and toxin extrusion proteins MATE1 (SLC47A1) and MATE2 (SLC47A2) and the plasma membrane monoamine transporter PMAT (SLC29A4/hENT4). Therefore, impacting variants in any of these transporters may have an influence in metformin efficacy and adverse effects (**Table 1**). In this context, the most studied genes are SLC22A1/OCT1, SLC22A2/OCT2, SLC47A1/MATE1 and SLC47A2/MATE2. Genetic variants in SLC22A1/OCT1 are responsible for the adverse gastrointestinal effects experienced by many patients with T2D diabetes who use metformin. Dujic et al. found that 47% of participants with T2D, incident users of metformin, experienced gastrointestinal adverse effects. In the study the number of SLC22A1/OCT1 reduced-function alleles was highly correlated with over two-fold risk of gastrointestinal side effect development [20]. Consequently, the gastrointestinal adverse effects and in some cases intolerance to metformin could lead to treatment abandonment. In this same gene other variants associated to metformin response have been reported. As it can be seen in **Table 1**, most of the reported variants are related to a decrease in the effect of metformin, reflected in the less reduction in HbA1c levels (high concentration of HbA1c). In contrast variant rs316019 in SLC22A2/OCT2 is associated with lactic acidosis and better response to metformin, due to the evidence that this variant is related to a reduced level of metformin clearance [30, 104]. Therefore, patients with these variants may benefit receiving alternative therapy instead metformin.

The studies that evaluated the role of SLC47A1/MATE1 and SLC47A2/MATE2 SNPs in PK and PD in patients receiving metformin revealed that promoter variants in MATE1 (g.-66 T → C, rs2252281; g.-130G → A, rs2289669) are associated with a greater response to the drug in T2D patients [34, 35]. Interestingly, it is also reported that the MATE1 variant affects the PD but not the PK of metformin, a very important finding that reveals that the distribution of drugs occurs in response to the organ-specific location of the various transporters [34]. Most studies have associated variants in SLC47A2/MATE2 with contradictory effects. Concerning rs12943590, it was related to a reduced response in European populations and a better metformin response in South Indian populations; whilst rs34399035 was associated with a reduced response to metformin in European populations [31, 34]. It is important to mention that the studies were carried out in different populations, and that investigations in other ethnicities had not found associations between these variants and metformin response [105, 106]. In a recent meta-analysis by Dujic et al. there was no association between rs12943590 and glycemic response [107]. Nonetheless, it is important to note that SNP-drug interactions and SNP-SNP interactions cannot be ruled out, since the presence of other SNPs also modulate the response to drugs and are different in each individual, thus, genotyping of these SNPs should be considered if it is desired apply personalized medicine in diseases such as T2D [34].

Other SNPs in candidate genes such as SLC2A2/GLUT2 (solute carrier family 2/Glucose transporter 2) have been associated with reduction in HbA1c or treatment success, together with rs11212617 in *C11orf65* (MFI, inhibitor of mitochondrial fission), in rs2162145 CPA6 (encoded protein CBPA6, this peptidase may convert inactive angiotensin I into the biologically active angiotensin II) and rs2162145 in STK11 (serine/threonine-protein kinase involved in cell metabolism) [36–39]. In contrast, variants in genes *PRPF31* (PRP31), CAPN10 (CAN10), SP1, FMO5 and *SLC22A3* (OCT3) are related to reduced response to metformin. Nonetheless, these associations have not been replicated in other studies or populations.

2.1.2 Sulfonylureas

Sulfonylureas are a class of oral antidiabetic agents widely used for the management of T2D [108]. They are chosen in the first line of treatment if the patient does not present with obesity or with insulin resistance or if there is intolerance or contraindication to metformin. Also, they are used in the second line in combination with other oral hypoglycemic agents, such as metformin [109]. According to the 2003–2016 National Health and Nutrition Examination Survey (NHANES), sulfonylurea monotherapy decreased from 33–8%, nonetheless, the combination with insulin or metformin was used in 50% of patients in the mentioned period [110]. Patients with a short duration of diabetes with residual beta cell function (high C-peptide levels) are likely to be most responsive to sulfonylurea therapy [111]. The mechanism of action of sulfonylureas consists of promoting insulin secretion via binding to sulfonylurea receptor 1 (SUR1), an element of the ATP-sensitive K+ (KATP) channel. The link between sulfonylurea and SUR1 inhibits the K-ATP channel, depolarizing the β cells, increasing intracellular Ca^{2+}, and consequently insulin granule exocytosis [112]. The rise of insulin levels regulates postprandial glycemia, stimulating peripheral glucose utilization [113]. Despite, sulfonylureas have a relatively short half-lifes (3 to 5 hours); they can cause hypoglycemia, which affects the quality of life and adherence to therapy in patients with T2D [114]. Two studies have reported hypoglycemia had occurred in 16–39% of patients treated with sulfonylureas [115, 116]. As a consequence, it has been estimated that 10–20% of individuals treated with sulfonylureas do not attain adequate glycemic control and 5–10% initially responding to sulfonylurea subsequently lose the ability to maintain normal glycemic level [117].

The most commonly used sulfonylureas, including the second-generation: glyburide, glipizide, and glimepiride are mainly metabolized through the cytochrome P450 (CYP) 2C9 enzyme. CYP2C9 belongs to the cytochrome P450 gene family and is the enzyme most abundantly expressed in liver. Indeed, CYP2C9 accounts for approximately 20% of total hepatic P450 protein, based on mass spectrometry quantitation [118]. It contributes to the metabolism of approximately 15% of all drugs that are subject to P450-catalyzed biotransformation, and it is responsible for >25% of metabolic clearance of oral hypoglycemic agents, such as chlorpropamide, glibenclamide, gliclazide, glimepiride, nateglinide and tolbutamide [119, 120]. Although CYP2C9 is highly polymorphic, however, only two polymorphisms have shown impact in enzyme expression and function, both allelic variants CYP2C9*2 (Arg144Cys, rs1799853) and CYP2C9*3 (Ile359Leu, rs1057910), encode proteins with less enzymatic activity for the metabolism of several substrates compared with the wild-type allele CYP2C9*1 (Arg144/Ile359). CYP2C9*2 and CYP2C9*3 are generally associated with more than 80% reduction in CYP2C9-mediated intrinsic clearance, while the effect of CYP2C9*2 is generally slightly smaller and varies considerably, depending on the substrate [120]. In both cases patients present more drug event reactions. Some studies have shown that CYP2C9 loss-of function alleles CYP2C9*2/*3 are associated with higher sulfonylurea levels and greater response to sulfonylureas. In the Go-DARTS study, patients with two copies of a loss-of-function allele were 3.4 times more probable to reach good glycemic control compared with patients with two wild-type CYP2C9 alleles, corresponding with a 0.5% greater reduction in HbA1c [44, 45]. In several pharmacokinetic studies the two variants rs1799853 and rs1057910 in CYP2C9 have been associated with hypoglycemic events, suggesting identification of these variants as a tool to predict adverse effects of these drugs in the patients with T2D [121].

Polymorphisms in KCNJ11, ABCC8, NOS1AP, TCF7L2, CYP2C8, KCNQ1, and IRS1 genes have been associated with altered therapeutic response to sulfonylureas, which will be described below [122]. ABCC8 and KCNJ11 encode K-ATP channel proteins SUR1 and Kir6.2, respectively, both form the K-ATP channel, which controls glucose-dependent insulin secretion in pancreatic β-cells [123, 124]. It has been reported that 50% of cases of neonatal diabetes are caused by mutations in KNJ11 or ABCC8 (SUR1) [125]. Therefore, genetic variants in ABCC8 and KCNJ11 genes could influence K-ATP channel function of beta cells, leading to changes in depolarization of the cell membrane and impact insulin secretion. Most studied SNPs in the ABCC8 gene include rs757110 (Ser1369Ala), rs1799854 (intronic variant) and rs1799859 (Arg1273Arg). Feng et al. demonstrated the association of the Ser1369Ala variant in the ABCC8 gene with fasting plasma glucose test (FPG) and two-hour plasma glucose after oral glucose tolerance test decreases after 8 weeks of gliclazide therapy. Additionally, the authors found a nominal association of the variant with levels of HbA1c, suggesting a role of this SNP on antidiabetic efficacy of gliclazides [46]. Several authors have attempted to associate this variant with insulin secretion; however, the findings have been contradictory. A study in the Diabetes Prevention Program population that includes Caucasian, African Americans, Hispanic Americans, American Indians and Asian Americans, found an association with a significantly lower insulin index, nevertheless, other studies failed to replicate this association [126–128]. Despite these data, it is interesting to mention that variant Ser1369Ala has been related with progression to diabetes [126]. Nikolac et al., found that rs1799854 and rs1799859 in the ABCC8 gene were associated with sulfonylurea efficacy in Caucasians, evidenced by significantly lower HbA1c concentrations in carriers compared with noncarriers [48].

As mentioned above, the KCNJ11 gene encodes the Kir6.2 subunit; four pore forming subunits assemble with four regulatory subunits of SUR1 to form the K-ATP channel of the β-cell [129]. Two SNPs have been associated with sulfonylureas response, rs5219 and rs5210. The rs5219 (Lys23Glu, p.E23K) A allele plays an important role in insulin secretion through reduction of ATP sensitivity of the K-ATP channel and suppression of insulin secretion. Previous studies, have demonstrated that carriers of a common variant, E23K, with normal glucose tolerance showed up to 40% reduction in glucose-stimulated insulin secretion [130, 131]. However, the mechanism of action of this locus in the insulin secretion pathway is still not completely understood. Although early observations have reported that E23K carriers exhibit higher predisposition to secondary failure when treated with sulfonylureas, other investigations have associated this variant with a better response to sulfonylureas [50, 51, 132, 133]. Additionally, some studies have suggested that the presence of the E23K variant is related to the severity of hypoglycemia in patients with sulfonylureas therapy or with lower response [52, 133]. Regarding rs5210, it has been reported that the G allele acts as a potential target for miR-1910, which is implicated in T2D; however, the mechanism of action of this miRNA in the development of T2D is unknown [134]. Moreover, variant rs5210, has been associated with gliclazide response, revealed by decreased levels of FPG test in carriers of this SNP [46].

The KCNQ1 gene belongs to a large family of voltage-gated K+ channels [135]. Although KCNQ1 is mainly expressed in the tissues or cells in the heart, it is also expressed in other tissues or organs such as pancreas islets [136]. Blockading the channels with KCNQ1 inhibitors, might stimulate secretion of insulin in pancreas, suggesting the association of KCNQ1 with the regulation of insulin secretion, specifically with reduced insulin secretion [137]. The intronic SNPs rs2237892 and rs2237895 were shown to increase gliclazide efficacy, whereas the intronic variant rs163184, was reported to lower-sulfonylureas effects on FPG levels [53, 54].

The transcription-factor-7-like-2 (TCF7L2) gene encodes the transcription factor 7 like-2 [138]. TCF7L2 can act through GLP-1 protein (Glucagon Like Peptide 1), which plays a central role in glucose homeostasis and is involved in the regulation of insulin secretion [139]. Several studies have suggested that TCF7L2 stimulates the proliferation of β-cells in the pancreas and facilitate the production of GLP-1 in intestinal cells. In this context, it is postulated that the SNP rs7903146 could decrease the expression levels of TCF7L2 in the pancreas and lead to lower secretion of insulin due to the decreased levels of GLP1. However, the association between TCF7L2 and T2D is more complex and is not limited to the decrease in GLP1, but also to alterations in other processes regulated by TCF7L2 such as the differentiation of pancreatic beta cells, in the normal metabolism of cholesterol and in the production of other incretins [140]. Pearson et al. determined the association of two genetic variants rs1225372 and rs7903146 in TCF7L2 with the treatment success of sulfonylurea therapy in T2D patients. It was shown that 12% of the diabetic population are homozygous carriers of SNP rs1225372 and were twice as unlikely to achieve good glycemic control within 1 year of treatment initiation compared to 42% of the population with wild type [56]. These findings were replicated in Indian and European populations among others [57, 141]. Therefore, carriers of these variants are at high risk of therapy failure with sulfonylureas.

The rest of SNPs that were associated with decreased response to sulfonylurea treatment and are found in the following genes: nitric oxide synthase 1 adaptor protein (NOS1AP), insulin receptor substrate 1 (IRS-1) and ATP binding cassette subfamily A member 1 (ABCA1). NOS1AP binds to neuronal nitric oxide synthase (nNOS). This enzyme plays a role in the electrical current of the heart and in insulin release from pancreatic β cells [142, 143]. Some polymorphisms in the NOS1AP gene have been described as predictive markers of cardiovascular mortality in diabetics treated with sulfonylureas. In patients with the rs10494366 TG/GG genotypes, glibenclamide is less effective in reducing glucose levels and mortality rates compared with the wild type TT genotype. By contrast, mortality risk was lower in tolbutamide and glimepiride users who carried a G allele compared with the T/T genotype [58]. Of note, no genotype differences in mortality were observed in metformin or insulin users. The mechanisms through which this polymorphism influenced mortality risk and the reason why this association differed based on the type of sulfonylurea used are unclear. Moreover, it was shown that in users of glibenclamide the TG and GG genotypes were associated with an increased risk of mortality; in tolbutamide and glimepiride users, the TG or GG genotypes were associated with a reduced risk of mortality [144]. Conversely, in a Korean study no significance was found between rs10494366 in the NOS1AP gene and response on glimepiride treatment [145].

Regarding rs1801278 in the ISR-1 gene, this variant has been associated with increased risk for secondary failure in African an European populations [59, 60]. In case of rs9282541, T2D patients carriers of variant needed a higher dose of glyburide in order to achieve the same glucose lowering effect that persons with the wild type variant [61].

2.1.3 Thiazolidinediones

Thiazolidinediones (TZDs) are pharmacologic agents that specifically treat insulin resistance. TZDs are effective at lowering HbA1c by ~1–1.25% on average [146]. Despite durability in action, TZDs show weight gain which has limited their clinical utility [147, 148]. For every 1% reduction in HbA1c, an estimated 2–3%

weight gain is reported [149]. TZDs are transported into the liver by OATP1B1 (encoded by *SLCO1B1* gene) and metabolized by CYP450 2C8 enzyme (encoded by *CYP2C8* gene) [150, 151]. The most studied variant allele in the CYP2C8 gene is CYP2C8*3, which comprises two linked polymorphisms at codon 139 and codon 399 (Arg139Lys; Lys399Arg) [152].

TZDs decrease insulin resistance directly through activation of peroxisome proliferator-activated receptors-γ (PPARγ) receptors, which facilitate differentiation of mesenchymal stem cells into adipocytes, promote lipogenesis in peripheral adipocytes, decrease hepatic and peripheral triglycerides, decrease activity of visceral adipocytes, and increase adiponectin. These primary effects of TZDs markedly ameliorate insulin resistance and decrease insulin requirements [153, 154]. Individuals differ in drug response, and ~ 20–30% of diabetic patients fail to respond to thiazolidinediones [155]. To date, numerous case–control studies have been conducted to identify the possible relationship between PPARG gene polymorphisms with the risk of T2D in various ethnic populations [156]. The most common variant is located at exon-2 of PPARG, rs1801282, and consists of a non-synonym change Pro12Ala. This substitution leads to a change in the structure of PPARγ protein, which in turn decreases the binding effect of target genes, and reducing transcriptional activity [157]. PPARγ is also the target of antidiabetic TZD drugs, which have a unique and powerful insulin-sensitizing effect [158].

2.1.4 DPP-4 inhibitors/GLP-1 receptor agonists

Dipeptidyl peptidase-4 inhibitors (DPP-4 inhibitors) are enzyme inhibitors that inhibit the enzyme dipeptidyl peptidase-4 (DPP-4). Inhibition of the DPP-4 enzyme prolongs and enhances the activity of incretins which play an important role in insulin secretion and blood glucose regulation [159]. DPP-4 is a 766 amino acid transmembrane glycoprotein, which is also known as adenosine deaminase or CD26, is a ubiquitously expressed glycoprotein of 110 kDa, which was first characterized by Hopsu-Havu and Glenner [160].

The DPP4 gene encodes a serine aminopeptidase enzyme, which inactivates GLP-1, GIP and other proteins via dipeptide cleavage of the N-terminal amino acid. Other DPP-4 substrates include peptides containing proline or alanine, such as growth factors, chemokines, neuropeptides, and vasoactive peptides [161].

Inhibitors of DPP-4 reversibly inhibit the hydrolysis of endogenous incretins, which increases plasma levels of GIP and GLP- 1, producing an increase in insulin response and a decrease in glucagon secretion. Therefore, the increase in the concentration of GLP-1 in plasma is the pharmacological effect of DPP-4 inhibitors, which increases insulin synthesis in β cells of the pancreas, stimulates the growth of these cells and prevents apoptosis [162]. Hence, DPP4 inhibition leads to greater exposure to incretins and therefore prolongs the half-life of insulin action. Because of this, DPP4 became a major target for the treatment of T2D [163].

However, it has recently been reported that some patients taking DPP-4 inhibitors are at increased risk of heart failure. It has been suggested that DPP-4 polymorphisms could potentially lead to a change in gene expression in renal cells in patients with T2D; these changes would be related to the renin-angiotensin-aldosterone system causing cardio-renal damage or myocardial hypertrophy, however further studies are needed to clarified the impact of these polymorphisms in DPP-4 inhibitors response [164].

2.1.5 SGLT-2 inhibitors

Sodium-glucose cotransporter inhibitors are adjunctive medications in the treatment of T2D. These drugs decrease HbA1c concentrations in diabetic patients, with few adverse effects seen to date. In a healthy adult, the kidneys filter approximately 180 g of glucose per day, this is almost entirely reabsorbed into the circulation and less than 1% of glucose is excreted in the urine filtered. This reabsorption is possible thanks to the action of a family of transmembrane proteins called sodium-glucose cotransporters (SGLT, sodium glucose co-transporter) [165]. So far, seven types of sodium-glucose transporters have been identified. Particularly, type 2 (SGLT2) is responsible for glucose renal reabsorption; and is mainly found in the epithelial cells of the proximal convoluted tubule.

Glycosuria, which was initially observed as an etiopathogenic component of some renal and urinary complications in patients with T2D, has been proposed as a means to lower glucose concentrations through the pharmacological use of SGLT2 inhibitors [166]. Some SGLT-2 inhibitors can be glucuronidated by UGT enzymes (UDP-glucuronosyltransferase), thereby polymorphisms like UGT1A9*3 allele (rs72551330), in the genes encoding these drug-metabolizing enzymes could potentially influence its response. Despite, higher values of area under the curve (AUC) of canaglifozina in carriers if UGT1A9*3, the studies have not found clinical implications [90, 91]. Recently Zimdahl et al. found that common genetic variants in the SLC5A2 gene do not affect diabetes-related metabolic traits and they do not have a clinically relevant impact on response to treatment with the SGLT2 inhibitor empagliflozin [167]. Nonetheless, a study in a Caucasian population showed that rs9934336 carriers presented increased 30-min glucose concentrations after oral glucose tolerance test [92]. Studies on these drugs are few, because SGLT2 inhibitors are relatively recent. Thus, the efficacy and safety evaluation of these drugs in various clinical settings has not yet been fully established.

2.2 Epigenetics

Despite, the major contribution in drug response can be attributed to genetic components, common genetic polymorphisms explain only less than half of this genetically encoded variability, thus it is important to address other factors of drug response, such as pharmacoepigenomics [168].

Pharmacoepigenomics combines the analysis of genetic variations and epigenetic modifications in an effort to advance personalized medicine [169]. Epigenetic modification refers to processes that modify DNA or chromatin structure in a manner that alters the level of expression of genes but not the DNA sequence itself. Chemical processes that fall into the realm of epigenetics include DNA methylation and post-translational modifications of histones such as the addition of methyl, phosphate, and acetyl groups. These modifications influence the overall chromatin structure and the availability of gene regulatory regions to transcription machinery [170].

On the other hand, regulatory processes involve molecules such as miRNas. Although miRNAs do not directly interact with DNA, they inhibit mRNA translation, therefore it is considered as having epigenetic effects [158].

Specific genes can be expressed or silenced depending on specific stimulators, such as hormone levels, dietary components or drug exposure, and can also accommodate gene-expression changes in response to gene–environment interactions [171]. Although, the cellular machinery responsible for the secretion of miRNA is not fully understood yet, it is recognized that miRNAs are packaged into microvesicles, exosomes, lipid drops and apoptotic bodies by a broad range of cell types and can be found in various types of body fluids, such as serum, plasma, and urine [172]. The miRNAs participate as negative regulators in post-transcriptional processes inhibiting mRNA translation or degrading the mRNA via the seed sequence region at the 5′ end of the miRNA, which allows the binding to its

3-´untranslated region (3 -UTR) of mRNA. miRNAs are estimated to affect approximately 30% of the process of protein coding genes [173]. A single miRNA is responsible for the expression of hundreds of proteins, and a protein-coding gene can be modulated by more than one miRNA, this is therefore a highly complex mechanism, but its results largely contribute to inter-individual variability in response to drugs. Although the study of miRNAs has focused on their involvement in the genesis of some complex diseases [174, 175] there is some evidence about their participation in the response to treatment in T2D. Interestingly the treatment with dapagliflozin (an inhibitor of sodium-glucose co-transporter 2, SGLT2), but not with hydrochlorothiazide (useful in treating high blood pressure), significantly up-regulated miR30e-5p and downregulated miR199a-3p ($P < 0.05$). These miRNAs are involved in the pathophysiology of heart failure and suggest a cardioprotective effect of SGLT2 inhibitor response [165].

Metformin can also interfere with the levels of miRNAs in the blood, which results in a change in the expression of the genes that are controlled by these. Ortega et al. have shown that increasing the dose of metformin modifies the levels of circulating miRNAs (started at a 425 mg/day and increased progressively during the first week to reach 1,700 mg/day), increased miR-192 (49.5%; $P = 0.022$) and decreased miR-140-5p (−15.8%; $P = 0.004$), and miR-222 (−47.2%; $P = 0.03$), in parallel to decreased fasting glucose and HbA1c. Revealing the response of circulating miRNAs to metformin therapy [95].

The information generated on miRNAs and their molecular actions place these molecules as innovative applications in the industry. Among the most promising prospects is the use of miRNA in medical therapy. Future studies of miRNAs that allow the generation of knowledge about their probable role in the modulation of pharmacogene expression will undoubtedly contribute to personalizing the treatment of T2D. miRNA-based therapies offer advantages over other nucleic acid therapies, because miRNAs are efficient silencers and, in contrast to plasmid DNA or synthetic oligonucleotides, miRNAs are naturally found in the bloodstream. As they target multiple mRNAs, the resulting synergistic effects could be positive for therapy, however, there are still multiple aspects that must be addressed before application to clinical trials in various human pathologies, among them, to identify the best miRNA candidates of miRNA targets for each disease type, the design of more efficient vehicles for the targeted delivery of oligonucleotides to specific organs, as well as avoiding potential toxicities and off-target effects. Low toxicity and good tolerance in patients treated with antagomiR a 15-nucleotide locked nucleic acid–modified antisense oligonucleotide whose action is sequestering mature miR-122 in a highly stable heteroduplex, thereby inhibiting its function avoiding the stability and propagation of hepatitis C virus (HCV), supporting the beneficial role of miRNAs in therapy [176]. miRNAs are naturally endogenous regulators of cell processes that are often dysregulated in diabetes restoration of any given miRNA function to normal levels will be the ultimate therapeutic goal. Several miRNAs appear to affect the function of the differentiated state of the pancreatic β-cell, while miRNAs in skeletal muscle, the liver, and adipose tissue constitute sets of different miRNAs, which is why the choice of the best molecules to treat this disease becomes very complex. Several challenges will need to be overcome in the field of pharmacotherapy with miRNA in the control of diabetes, but they will undoubtedly contribute to personalizing the treatment of this disease.

It has been suggested that epigenomics may act synergistically with pharmacogenomics towards optimization of drug therapy [177]. In addition, epigenomic somatic alterations represent an emerging class of biomarkers that hold promise for personalized therapy particularly to overcome drug resistance [178].

Regarding methylation, García-Calzón et al. evaluated the potential blood epigenetic markers associated with metformin glycemic and intolerance response. They analyzed DNA methylation in blood from newly diagnosed patients with T2D after 1.5 years of metformin treatment. According to the authors, the methylation risk scores explain 68–73% of the variation in glycemic response to metformin. In addition, the methylation risk scores explain 50–51% of the variation in metformin tolerance. In the same study, the researchers also assessed whether any of 26 SNPs previously associated with metformin response were associated with DNA methylation of any of the identified epigenetic markers. They identified one significant association between a SNP in SCL22A1 (rs628031) and DNA methylation of cg05151280 ($P = 0.001$, $q = 0.028$). The A/A genotype carriers had lower methylation ($83.6 \pm 2.3\%$) compared to carriers of the G/G ($85.3 \pm 1.9\%$, $P = 0.002$) and G/A ($85 \pm 1.8\%$, $P = 0.006$) genotypes in 132 participants from the discovery and replication cohorts. Lower methylation of this CpG site was associated with a better glycemic response to metformin (**Table 2**) [93]. In previous work from the same group, they assessed the DNA methylation in OCT1 encoded by *SLC22A1*, OCT3 encoded by *SLC22A3*, and MATE1 encoded by *SLC47A1* liver biopsies from gastric bypass surgery. Lower promoter DNA methylation of *SLC22A1*, *SLC22A3*, and *SLC47A1* were found in diabetic subjects receiving metformin. These findings suggest that metformin decreases DNA methylation of metformin transporter genes in the human liver, in contrast with the higher methylation levels in these genes associated with hyperglycemia and obesity. These findings show how a drug is capable of modulating gene expression however, the presence of genetic variants in these genes would be interfering with the methylation process with unexpected results [94].

Methylation in KCNJ11 and ABCC8 gene promoters in T2D patients receiving sulfonylurea therapy have been assessed by Karaglani et al., their results show that epigenetic changes such as methylation influence interindividual variability in treatment with sulfonylureas. They considered hypoglycemia as an outcome of the treatment. KCNJ11 methylation was detected in 21.6% of hypoglycemic individuals and in 27.7% of non-hypoglycemic patients ($P = 0.353$) in this study, while ABCC8 methylation in 7.2% of non-hypoglycemic and none of the hypoglycemic patients ($P = 0.012$). These findings suggest that ABCC8 methylation is associated with hypoglycemic events in sulfonylurea-treated T2D patients [97].

3. Conclusions

The interindividual variability in the response to a drug is the consequence of various factors, including pharmacokinetic causes: absorption, distribution, metabolization and excretion of the drug that affects the intensity and duration of the response, or to pharmacodynamic causes in drug-receptor interaction. Each of these PK and PD factors is different in each individual due to genetic, environmental or pathological determinants, and also depends on the severity or intensity of the disease to be treated.

One of the main obstacles to transferring findings from pharmacogenetics to the clinic is the impact of ethnicity on genetic variation. The highly significant associations between SNPs and the response modulated by pharmacogenetics can differ considerably between populations, which has a direct impact on drug use and dosage decisions. It is necessary then that the studies to evaluate pharmacological efficacy and pharmacogenetics, have uniformity in research designs, dosage regimens, study populations, and analytical methods.

The epidemic of T2D has forced the use of drugs that aim at glycemic control and avoid secondary complications that cause very high medical costs and decrease the quality of life of patients. However, it has been observed that even though many patients carefully follow medical guidelines, the glycemic control so desired is not achieved. Thus, with the advent of pharmacogenomics, various studies are carried out to achieve personalized medicine in this field having an impact on a better quality of life and also reducing the costs of treatment of this disease by the Health services.

In this review, the main drugs used for the treatment of T2D were analyzed and the implications that the various SNPs have on their target genes, which will affect their pharmacological response. All this opens the way for us to apply these genomic findings in daily clinical practice, in search of personalized medicine that impacts adequate glycemic control in patients with T2D in search of a better quality of life.

Author details

Katy Sánchez-Pozos[1], María de los Ángeles Granados-Silvestre[2] and María Guadalupe Ortíz-López[1]*

1 Laboratory of Molecular Endocrinology, Hospital Juárez de México, Mexico City, Mexico

2 Laboratory of Diabetes, Facultad de Química, Universidad Nacional Autónoma de México, Mexico City, Mexico

*Address all correspondence to: gortizl@prodigy.net.mx

References

[1] Kalow W, Endrenyi L, Tang B. Repeat administration of drugs as a means to assess the genetic component in pharmacological variability. Pharmacology. 1999 Jun;58(6):281–4.

[2] Gamazon ER, Perera M. Genome-wide approaches in pharmacogenomics: heritability estimation and pharmacoethnicity as primary challenges. Vol. 13, Pharmacogenomics. 2012. p. 1101–4.

[3] Vesell ES. Genetic and environmental factors causing variation in drug response. Vol. 247, Mutation Research. 1991.

[4] Rasmussen BB, Brix TH, Kyvik KO, Brøsen K. The interindividual differences in the 3-demthylation of caffeine alias CYP1A2 is determined by both genetic and environmental factors. Pharmacogenetics. 2002 Aug;12(6): 473–8.

[5] Matthaei J, Tzvetkov M V, Strube J, Sehrt D, Sachse-Seeboth C, Hjelmborg JB, et al. Heritability of Caffeine Metabolism: Environmental Effects Masking Genetic Effects on CYP1A2 Activity but Not on NAT2. Clin Pharmacol Ther. 2016 Dec;100(6): 606–16.

[6] Matthaei J, Brockmöller J, Tzvetkov M V, Sehrt D, Sachse-Seeboth C, Hjelmborg JB, et al. Heritability of metoprolol and torsemide pharmacokinetics. Clin Pharmacol Ther. 2015 Dec;98(6):611–21.

[7] Matthaei J, Tzvetkov M V, Gal V, Sachse-Seeboth C, Sehrt D, Hjelmborg JB, et al. Low heritability in pharmacokinetics of talinolol: a pharmacogenetic twin study on the heritability of the pharmacokinetics of talinolol, a putative probe drug of MDR1 and other membrane transporters. Genome Med. 2016 Nov;8(1):119.

[8] Jensen O, Matthaei J, Blome F, Schwab M, Tzvetkov M V, Brockmöller J. Variability and Heritability of Thiamine Pharmacokinetics With Focus on OCT1 Effects on Membrane Transport and Pharmacokinetics in Humans. Clin Pharmacol Ther. 2020 Mar;107(3): 628–38.

[9] Scott J, Poffenbarger PL. Pharmacogenetics of tolbutamide metabolism in humans. Diabetes. 1979 Jan;28(1):41–51.

[10] Gjesing AP, Hornbak M, Allin KH, Ekstrøm CT, Urhammer SA, Eiberg H, et al. High heritability and genetic correlation of intravenous glucose- and tolbutamide-induced insulin secretion among non-diabetic family members of type 2 diabetic patients. Diabetologia. 2014 Jun;57(6):1173–81.

[11] Zhou K, Donnelly L, Yang J, Li M, Deshmukh H, Van Zuydam N, et al. Heritability of variation in glycaemic response to metformin: a genome-wide complex trait analysis. lancet Diabetes Endocrinol. 2014 Jun;2(6):481–7.

[12] Online version IDF Diabetes Atlas [Internet]. [cited 2020 Dec 17]. Available from: www.diabetesatlas.org

[13] Diagnosis and classification of diabetes mellitus. Diabetes Care. 2009 Jan;32 Suppl 1(Suppl 1):S62-7.

[14] Lorenzoni V, Baccetti F, Genovese S, Torre E, Turchetti G. Cost-consequence analysis of sitagliptin versus sulfonylureas as add-on therapy for the treatment of diabetic patients in Italy. Clinicoecon Outcomes Res. 2017;9: 699–710.

[15] Cowie CC. Diabetes Diagnosis and Control: Missed Opportunities to Improve Health. Diabetes Care [Internet]. 2019 Jun 1;42(6):994 LP

– 1004. Available from: http://care.diabetesjournals.org/content/42/6/994.abstract

[16] Shrestha J, Prajapati M, Karkee A, Shrestha H, Maharjan A. Adverse Effects of Oral Hypoglycemic Agents and Adherence to them among Patients with Type 2 Diabetes Mellitus in Nepal. J Lumbini Med Coll. 2017 Jun 29;5:6.

[17] Chahal H. Oral hypoglycemics (Review) – Adults. 19th Expert Committee on the Selection and Use of Essential Medicines. 2013.

[18] Edridge CL, Dunkley AJ, Bodicoat DH, Rose TC, Gray LJ, Davies MJ, et al. Prevalence and Incidence of Hypoglycaemia in 532,542 People with Type 2 Diabetes on Oral Therapies and Insulin: A Systematic Review and Meta-Analysis of Population Based Studies. PLoS One. 2015;10(6):e0126427.

[19] Mannino GC, Andreozzi F, Sesti G. Pharmacogenetics of type 2 diabetes mellitus, the route toward tailored medicine. Diabetes Metab Res Rev. 2019 Mar;35(3):e3109.

[20] Dujic T, Causevic A, Bego T, Malenica M, Velija-Asimi Z, Pearson ER, et al. Organic cation transporter 1 variants and gastrointestinal side effects of metformin in patients with Type 2 diabetes. Diabet Med [Internet]. 2016; 33(4):511–4. Available from: https://onlinelibrary.wiley.com/doi/abs/10.1111/dme.13040

[21] Dujic T, Zhou K, Donnelly LA, Tavendale R, Palmer CNA, Pearson ER. Association of Organic Cation Transporter 1 With Intolerance to Metformin in Type 2 Diabetes: A GoDARTS Study. Diabetes [Internet]. 2015 May 1;64(5):1786 LP – 1793. Available from: http://diabetes.diabetesjournals.org/content/64/5/1786.abstract

[22] Christensen MMH, Brasch-Andersen C, Green H, Nielsen F, Damkier P, Beck-Nielsen H, et al. The pharmacogenetics of metformin and its impact on plasma metformin steady-state levels and glycosylated hemoglobin A1c. Pharmacogenet Genomics. 2011 Dec;21(12):837–50.

[23] Zhou Y, Ye W, Wang Y, Jiang Z, Meng X, Xiao Q, et al. Genetic variants of OCT1 influence glycemic response to metformin in Han Chinese patients with type-2 diabetes mellitus in Shanghai. Int J Clin Exp Pathol. 2015;8(8):9533–42.

[24] Umamaheswaran G, Praveen RG, Damodaran SE, Das AK, Adithan C. Influence of SLC22A1 rs622342 genetic polymorphism on metformin response in South Indian type 2 diabetes mellitus patients. Clin Exp Med. 2015 Nov;15(4):511–7.

[25] Becker ML, Visser LE, van Schaik RHN, Hofman A, Uitterlinden AG, Stricker BHC. Genetic variation in the organic cation transporter 1 is associated with metformin response in patients with diabetes mellitus. Pharmacogenomics J. 2009 Aug;9(4):242–7.

[26] Reséndiz-Abarca CA, Flores-Alfaro E, Suárez-Sánchez F, Cruz M, Valladares-Salgado A, Del Carmen Alarcón-Romero L, et al. Altered Glycemic Control Associated With Polymorphisms in the SLC22A1 (OCT1) Gene in a Mexican Population With Type 2 Diabetes Mellitus Treated With Metformin: A Cohort Study. J Clin Pharmacol. 2019 Oct;59(10):1384–90.

[27] Tarasova L, Kalnina I, Geldnere K, Bumbure A, Ritenberga R, Nikitina-Zake L, et al. Association of genetic variation in the organic cation transporters OCT1, OCT2 and multidrug and toxin extrusion 1 transporter protein genes with the gastrointestinal side effects and lower

BMI in metformin-treated type 2 diabetes patients. Pharmacogenet Genomics. 2012 Sep;22(9):659–66.

[28] Xiao D, Guo Y, Li X, Yin J-Y, Zheng W, Qiu X-W, et al. The Impacts of SLC22A1 rs594709 and SLC47A1 rs2289669 Polymorphisms on Metformin Therapeutic Efficacy in Chinese Type 2 Diabetes Patients. Int J Endocrinol. 2016;2016:4350712.

[29] Kashi Z, Masoumi P, Mahrooz A, Hashemi-Soteh MB, Bahar A, Alizadeh A. The variant organic cation transporter 2 (OCT2)-T201M contribute to changes in insulin resistance in patients with type 2 diabetes treated with metformin. Diabetes Res Clin Pract. 2015 Apr;108(1):78–83.

[30] Li Q, Liu F, Zheng T, Tang J, Lu H, Jia W. SLC22A2 gene 808 G/T variant is related to plasma lactate concentration in Chinese type 2 diabetics treated with metformin. Acta Pharmacol Sin. 2010 Feb;31(2):184–90.

[31] Phani NM, Vohra M, Kakar A, Adhikari P, Nagri SK, D'Souza SC, et al. Implication of critical pharmacokinetic gene variants on therapeutic response to metformin in Type 2 diabetes. Pharmacogenomics. 2018 Jul;19(11): 905–11.

[32] Li Q, Li C, Li H, Zeng L, Kang Z, Mao Y, et al. STK11 rs2075604 Polymorphism Is Associated with Metformin Efficacy in Chinese Type 2 Diabetes Mellitus. Int J Endocrinol. 2017;2017:3402808.

[33] Zaharenko L, Kalnina I, Geldnere K, Konrade I, Grinberga S, Židzik J, et al. Single nucleotide polymorphisms in the intergenic region between metformin transporter OCT2 and OCT3 coding genes are associated with short-term response to metformin monotherapy in type 2 diabetes mellitus patients. Eur J Endocrinol. 2016 Dec;175(6): 531–40.

[34] Stocker SL, Morrissey KM, Yee SW, Castro RA, Xu L, Dahlin A, et al. The effect of novel promoter variants in MATE1 and MATE2 on the pharmacokinetics and pharmacodynamics of metformin. Clin Pharmacol Ther. 2013 Feb;93(2):186–94.

[35] Tkáč I, Klimčáková L, Javorský M, Fabianová M, Schroner Z, Hermanová H, et al. Pharmacogenomic association between a variant in SLC47A1 gene and therapeutic response to metformin in type 2 diabetes. Diabetes Obes Metab. 2013 Feb;15(2): 189–91.

[36] Zhou K, Yee SW, Seiser EL, van Leeuwen N, Tavendale R, Bennett AJ, et al. Variation in the glucose transporter gene SLC2A2 is associated with glycemic response to metformin. Nat Genet. 2016 Sep;48(9):1055–9.

[37] Rathmann W, Strassburger K, Bongaerts B, Kuss O, Müssig K, Burkart V, et al. A variant of the glucose transporter gene SLC2A2 modifies the glycaemic response to metformin therapy in recently diagnosed type 2 diabetes. Diabetologia. 2019 Feb;62(2): 286–91.

[38] van Leeuwen N, Nijpels G, Becker ML, Deshmukh H, Zhou K, Stricker BHC, et al. A gene variant near ATM is significantly associated with metformin treatment response in type 2 diabetes: a replication and meta-analysis of five cohorts. Diabetologia. 2012 Jul;55 (7):1971–7.

[39] Rotroff DM, Yee SW, Zhou K, Marvel SW, Shah HS, Jack JR, et al. Genetic Variants in CPA6 and PRPF31 Are Associated With Variation in Response to Metformin in Individuals With Type 2 Diabetes. Diabetes. 2018 Jul;67(7):1428–40.

[40] Tkáč I, Javorský M, Klimčáková L, Židzik J, Gaľa I, Babjaková E, et al. A pharmacogenetic association between a

variation in calpain 10 (CAPN10) gene and the response to metformin treatment in patients with type 2 diabetes. Eur J Clin Pharmacol. 2015 Jan; 71(1):59–63.

[41] Goswami S, Yee SW, Stocker S, Mosley JD, Kubo M, Castro R, et al. Genetic variants in transcription factors are associated with the pharmacokinetics and pharmacodynamics of metformin. Clin Pharmacol Ther. 2014 Sep;96(3):370–9.

[42] Breitenstein MK, Wang L, Simon G, Ryu E, Armasu SM, Ray B, et al. Leveraging an Electronic Health Record-Linked Biorepository to Generate a Metformin Pharmacogenomics Hypothesis. AMIA Jt Summits Transl Sci proceedings AMIA Jt Summits Transl Sci. 2015;2015: 26–30.

[43] Chen EC, Liang X, Yee SW, Geier EG, Stocker SL, Chen L, et al. Targeted disruption of organic cation transporter 3 attenuates the pharmacologic response to metformin. Mol Pharmacol. 2015 Jul;88(1):75–83.

[44] Zhou K, Donnelly L, Burch L, Tavendale R, Doney ASF, Leese G, et al. Loss-of-function CYP2C9 variants improve therapeutic response to sulfonylureas in type 2 diabetes: a Go-DARTS study. Clin Pharmacol Ther. 2010 Jan;87(1):52–6.

[45] Castelán-Martínez OD, Hoyo-Vadillo C, Bazán-Soto TB, Cruz M, Tesoro-Cruz E, Valladares-Salgado A. CYP2C9*3 gene variant contributes independently to glycaemic control in patients with type 2 diabetes treated with glibenclamide. J Clin Pharm Ther. 2018 Dec;43(6):768–74.

[46] Feng Y, Mao G, Ren X, Xing H, Tang G, Li Q, et al. Ser1369Ala variant in sulfonylurea receptor gene ABCC8 is associated with antidiabetic efficacy of gliclazide in Chinese type 2 diabetic patients. Diabetes Care. 2008 Oct;31 (10):1939–44.

[47] Zhang H, Liu X, Kuang H, Yi R, Xing H. Association of sulfonylurea receptor 1 genotype with therapeutic response to gliclazide in type 2 diabetes. Diabetes Res Clin Pract. 2007 Jul;77(1): 58–61.

[48] Nikolac N, Simundic A-M, Katalinic D, Topic E, Cipak A, Zjacic Rotkvic V. Metabolic control in type 2 diabetes is associated with sulfonylurea receptor-1 (SUR-1) but not with KCNJ11 polymorphisms. Arch Med Res. 2009 Jul;40(5):387–92.

[49] Zhou X, Chen C, Yin D, Zhao F, Bao Z, Zhao Y, et al. A Variation in the ABCC8 Gene Is Associated with Type 2 Diabetes Mellitus and Repaglinide Efficacy in Chinese Type 2 Diabetes Mellitus Patients. Intern Med. 2019 Aug; 58(16):2341–7.

[50] Javorsky M, Klimcakova L, Schroner Z, Zidzik J, Babjakova E, Fabianova M, et al. KCNJ11 gene E23K variant and therapeutic response to sulfonylureas. Eur J Intern Med. 2012 Apr;23(3):245–9.

[51] Li Q, Chen M, Zhang R, Jiang F, Wang J, Zhou J, et al. KCNJ11 E23K variant is associated with the therapeutic effect of sulphonylureas in Chinese type 2 diabetic patients. Clin Exp Pharmacol Physiol. 2014 Oct;41 (10):748–54.

[52] Sanchez-Ibarra HE, Reyes-Cortes LM, Jiang X-L, Luna-Aguirre CM, Aguirre-Trevino D, Morales-Alvarado IA, et al. Genotypic and Phenotypic Factors Influencing Drug Response in Mexican Patients With Type 2 Diabetes Mellitus. Front Pharmacol. 2018;9:320.

[53] Schroner Z, Dobrikova M, Klimcakova L, Javorsky M, Zidzik J, Kozarova M, et al. Variation in KCNQ1 is associated with therapeutic response

to sulphonylureas. Med Sci Monit Int Med J Exp Clin Res. 2011 Jul;17(7): CR392-6.

[54] Li Q, Tang T-T, Jiang F, Zhang R, Chen M, Yin J, et al. Polymorphisms of the KCNQ1 gene are associated with the therapeutic responses of sulfonylureas in Chinese patients with type 2 diabetes. Acta Pharmacol Sin. 2017 Jan;38(1): 80–9.

[55] Javorský M, Babjaková E, Klimčáková L, Schroner Z, Zidzik J, Stolfová M, et al. Association between TCF7L2 Genotype and Glycemic Control in Diabetic Patients Treated with Gliclazide. Int J Endocrinol. 2013; 2013:374858.

[56] Pearson ER, Donnelly LA, Kimber C, Whitley A, Doney ASF, McCarthy MI, et al. Variation in TCF7L2 influences therapeutic response to sulfonylureas: a GoDARTs study. Diabetes. 2007 Aug;56(8):2178–82.

[57] Holstein A, Hahn M, Körner A, Stumvoll M, Kovacs P. TCF7L2 and therapeutic response to sulfonylureas in patients with type 2 diabetes. BMC Med Genet. 2011 Feb;12:30.

[58] Becker ML, Aarnoudse A-JLHJ, Newton-Cheh C, Hofman A, Witteman JCM, Uitterlinden AG, et al. Common variation in the NOS1AP gene is associated with reduced glucose-lowering effect and with increased mortality in users of sulfonylurea. Pharmacogenet Genomics. 2008 Jul;18(7):591–7.

[59] El-Sisi AE, Hegazy SK, Metwally SS, Wafa AM, Dawood NA. Effect of genetic polymorphisms on the development of secondary failure to sulfonylurea in egyptian patients with type 2 diabetes. Ther Adv Endocrinol Metab. 2011 Aug;2(4):155–64.

[60] Sesti G, Marini MA, Cardellini M, Sciacqua A, Frontoni S, Andreozzi F, et al. The Arg972 variant in insulin receptor substrate-1 is associated with an increased risk of secondary failure to sulfonylurea in patients with type 2 diabetes. Diabetes Care. 2004 Jun;27(6): 1394–8.

[61] Aguilar-Salinas CA, Muñoz-Hernandez LL, Cobos-Bonilla M, Ramírez-Márquez MR, Ordoñez-Sanchez ML, Mehta R, et al. The R230C variant of the ATP binding cassette protein A1 (ABCA1) gene is associated with a decreased response to glyburide therapy in patients with type 2 diabetes mellitus. Metabolism. 2013 May;62(5): 638–41.

[62] Hsieh M-C, Lin K-D, Tien K-J, Tu S-T, Hsiao J-Y, Chang S-J, et al. Common polymorphisms of the peroxisome proliferator-activated receptor-gamma (Pro12Ala) and peroxisome proliferator-activated receptor-gamma coactivator-1 (Gly482Ser) and the response to pioglitazone in Chinese patients with type 2 diabetes mellitus. Metabolism. 2010 Aug;59(8):1139–44.

[63] Pei Q, Huang Q, Yang G, Zhao Y, Yin J, Song M, et al. PPAR-γ2 and PTPRD gene polymorphisms influence type 2 diabetes patients' response to pioglitazone in China. Acta Pharmacol Sin. 2013 Feb;34(2):255–61.

[64] Wolford JK, Yeatts KA, Dhanjal SK, Black MH, Xiang AH, Buchanan TA, et al. Sequence Variation in PPARG May Underlie Differential Response to Troglitazone. Diabetes [Internet]. 2005; 54(11):3319–25. Available from: https://diabetes.diabetesjournals.org/content/54/11/3319

[65] Zhang K-H, Huang Q, Dai X-P, Yin J-Y, Zhang W, Zhou G, et al. Effects of the peroxisome proliferator activated receptor-γ coactivator-1α (PGC-1α) Thr394Thr and Gly482Ser polymorphisms on rosiglitazone response in Chinese patients with type 2 diabetes mellitus. J Clin Pharmacol. 2010 Sep;50(9):1022–30.

[66] Yang M, Huang Q, Wu J, Yin J-Y, Sun H, Liu H-L, et al. Effects of UCP2-866 G/A and ADRB3 Trp64Arg on rosiglitazone response in Chinese patients with Type 2 diabetes. Br J Clin Pharmacol. 2009 Jul;68(1):14–22.

[67] Dawed AY, Donnelly L, Tavendale R, Carr F, Leese G, Palmer CNA, et al. CYP2C8 and SLCO1B1 Variants and Therapeutic Response to Thiazolidinediones in Patients With Type 2 Diabetes. Diabetes Care. 2016 Nov;39(11):1902–8.

[68] Sun H, Gong Z-C, Yin J-Y, Liu H-L, Liu Y-Z, Guo Z-W, et al. The association of adiponectin allele 45T/G and −11377C/G polymorphisms with Type 2 diabetes and rosiglitazone response in Chinese patients. Br J Clin Pharmacol. 2008;65(6):917–26.

[69] Yang H, Ye E, Si G, Chen L, Cai L, Ye C, et al. Adiponectin gene polymorphism rs2241766 T/G is associated with response to pioglitazone treatment in type 2 diabetic patients from southern China. PLoS One. 2014;9 (11):e112480.

[70] Kang ES, Park SY, Kim HJ, Ahn CW, Nam M, Cha BS, et al. The influence of adiponectin gene polymorphism on the rosiglitazone response in patients with type 2 diabetes. Diabetes Care. 2005 May;28 (5):1139–44.

[71] Li Z, Peng X, Wu Y, Xia Y, Liu X, Zhang Q. The influence of adiponectin gene polymorphism on the pioglitazone response in the Chinese with type 2 diabetes. Vol. 10, Diabetes, obesity & metabolism. England; 2008. p. 794–802.

[72] MAKINO H, SHIMIZU I, MURAO S, KONDO S, TABARA Y, FUJIYAMA M, et al. A Pilot Study Suggests that the G/G Genotype of Resistin Single Nucleotide Polymorphism at -420 May Be an Independent Predictor of a Reduction in Fasting Plasma Glucose and Insulin Resistance by Pioglitazone in Type 2 Diabetes. Endocr J. 2009;56 (9):1049–58.

[73] Liu H-L, Lin Y-G, Wu J, Sun H, Gong Z-C, Hu P-C, et al. Impact of genetic polymorphisms of leptin and TNF-alpha on rosiglitazone response in Chinese patients with type 2 diabetes. Eur J Clin Pharmacol. 2008 Jul;64(7): 663–71.

[74] Zimdahl H, Ittrich C, Graefe-Mody U, Boehm BO, Mark M, Woerle H-J, et al. Influence of TCF7L2 gene variants on the therapeutic response to the dipeptidylpeptidase-4 inhibitor linagliptin. Diabetologia. 2014 Sep;57 (9):1869–75.

[75] Jamaluddin JL, Huri HZ, Vethakkan SR. Clinical and genetic predictors of dipeptidyl peptidase-4 inhibitor treatment response in Type 2 diabetes mellitus. Pharmacogenomics. 2016 Jun;17(8):867–81.

[76] 't Hart LM, Fritsche A, Nijpels G, van Leeuwen N, Donnelly LA, Dekker JM, et al. The CTRB1/2 locus affects diabetes susceptibility and treatment via the incretin pathway. Diabetes. 2013 Sep;62(9):3275–81.

[77] Gotthardová I, Javorský M, Klimčáková L, Kvapil M, Schroner Z, Kozárová M, et al. KCNQ1 gene polymorphism is associated with glycaemic response to treatment with DPP-4 inhibitors. Diabetes Res Clin Pract. 2017 Aug;130:142–7.

[78] Han E, Park HS, Kwon O, Choe EY, Wang HJ, Lee Y-H, et al. A genetic variant in GLP1R is associated with response to DPP-4 inhibitors in patients with type 2 diabetes. Medicine (Baltimore). 2016 Nov;95(44):e5155.

[79] Javorský M, Gotthardová I, Klimčáková L, Kvapil M, Židzik J, Schroner Z, et al. A missense variant in

GLP1R gene is associated with the glycaemic response to treatment with gliptins. Diabetes Obes Metab. 2016 Sep; 18(9):941–4.

[80] Űrgeová A, Javorský M, Klimčáková L, Židzik J, Šalagovič J, Hubáček JA, et al. Genetic variants associated with glycemic response to treatment with dipeptidylpeptidase 4 inhibitors. Pharmacogenomics. 2020 Apr;21(5):317–23.

[81] Wilson JR, Shuey MM, Brown NJ, Devin JK. Hypertension and Type 2 Diabetes Are Associated With Decreased Inhibition of Dipeptidyl Peptidase-4 by Sitagliptin. J Endocr Soc. 2017 Sep;1(9):1168–78.

[82] Liao W-L, Lee W-J, Chen C-C, Lu CH, Chen C-H, Chou Y-C, et al. Pharmacogenetics of dipeptidyl peptidase 4 inhibitors in a Taiwanese population with type 2 diabetes. Oncotarget. 2017 Mar;8(11):18050–8.

[83] Iskakova A, Aitkulova A, Sikhayeva N, Romanova AA, Maratkyzy L, Akanov Z, et al. Dipeptidyl peptidase-4 inhibitors: sensitivity markers. Biotechnol Theory Pract. 2017 Sep 18;13–20.

[84] Osada UN, Sunagawa H, Terauchi Y, Ueda S. A Common Susceptibility Gene for Type 2 Diabetes Is Associated with Drug Response to a DPP-4 Inhibitor: Pharmacogenomic Cohort in Okinawa Japan. PLoS One. 2016;11(5):e0154821.

[85] Yu M, Wang K, Liu H, Cao R. GLP1R variant is associated with response to exenatide in overweight Chinese Type 2 diabetes patients. Pharmacogenomics. 2019 Mar;20(4): 273–7.

[86] Ferreira MC, da Silva MER, Fukui RT, do Carmo Arruda-Marques M, Azhar S, Dos Santos RF. Effect of TCF7L2 polymorphism on pancreatic hormones after exenatide in type 2 diabetes. Diabetol Metab Syndr. 2019;11:10.

[87] Lin C-H, Lee Y-S, Huang Y-Y, Hsieh S-H, Chen Z-S, Tsai C-N. Polymorphisms of GLP-1 receptor gene and response to GLP-1 analogue in patients with poorly controlled type 2 diabetes. J Diabetes Res. 2015;2015: 176949.

[88] Zhou LM, Xu W, Yan XM, Li MXY, Liang H, Weng JP. [Association between SORCS1 rs1416406 and therapeutic effect of exenatide]. Zhonghua Yi Xue Za Zhi. 2017 May;97(18):1415–9.

[89] de Luis DA, Aller R, Izaola O, de la Fuente B, Romero E. Genetic variation in the beta-3-adrenoreceptor gene (Trp64Arg polymorphism) and their influence on anthropometric parameters and insulin resistance after a high protein/low carbohydrate versus a standard hypocaloric diet. Nutr Hosp. 2015 Aug;32(2):487–93.

[90] Francke S, Mamidi RNVS, Solanki B, Scheers E, Jadwin A, Favis R, et al. In vitro metabolism of canagliflozin in human liver, kidney, intestine microsomes, and recombinant uridine diphosphate glucuronosyltransferases (UGT) and the effect of genetic variability of UGT enzymes on the pharmacokinetics of canagliflozin in humans. J Clin Pharmacol. 2015 Sep;55(9):1061–72.

[91] Hoeben E, De Winter W, Neyens M, Devineni D, Vermeulen A, Dunne A. Population Pharmacokinetic Modeling of Canagliflozin in Healthy Volunteers and Patients with Type 2 Diabetes Mellitus. Clin Pharmacokinet. 2016 Feb; 55(2):209–23.

[92] Enigk U, Breitfeld J, Schleinitz D, Dietrich K, Halbritter J, Fischer-Rosinsky A, et al. Role of genetic variation in the human sodium-glucose cotransporter 2 gene (SGLT2) in glucose

homeostasis. Pharmacogenomics. 2011 Aug;12(8):1119–26.

[93] García-Calzón S, Perfilyev A, Martinell M, Ustinova M, Kalamajski S, Franks PW, et al. Epigenetic markers associated with metformin response and intolerance in drug-naïve patients with type 2 diabetes. Sci Transl Med. 2020 Sep;12(561).

[94] García-Calzón S, Perfilyev A, Männistö V, de Mello VD, Nilsson E, Pihlajamäki J, et al. Diabetes medication associates with DNA methylation of metformin transporter genes in the human liver. Clin Epigenetics. 2017;9:102.

[95] Ortega FJ, Mercader JM, Moreno-Navarrete JM, Rovira O, Guerra E, Esteve E, et al. Profiling of circulating microRNAs reveals common microRNAs linked to type 2 diabetes that change with insulin sensitization. Diabetes Care. 2014;37(5):1375–83.

[96] Coleman CB, Lightell DJJ, Moss SC, Bates M, Parrino PE, Woods TC. Elevation of miR-221 and -222 in the internal mammary arteries of diabetic subjects and normalization with metformin. Mol Cell Endocrinol. 2013 Jul;374(1–2):125–9.

[97] Karaglani M, Ragia G, Panagopoulou M, Balgkouranidou I, Nena E, Kolios G, et al. Search for Pharmacoepigenetic Correlations in Type 2 Diabetes Under Sulfonylurea Treatment. Exp Clin Endocrinol diabetes Off journal, Ger Soc Endocrinol [and] Ger Diabetes Assoc. 2019 Apr;127(4):226–33.

[98] Solini A, Seghieri M, Giannini L, Biancalana E, Parolini F, Rossi C, et al. The Effects of Dapagliflozin on Systemic and Renal Vascular Function Display an Epigenetic Signature. J Clin Endocrinol Metab. 2019;104(10):4253–63.

[99] Shastry BS. SNPs: impact on gene function and phenotype. Methods Mol Biol. 2009;578:3–22.

[100] 9. Pharmacologic Approaches to Glycemic Treatment: Standards of Medical Care in Diabetes—2021. Diabetes Care. 2021 Jan;44(Supplement 1):S111 LP-S124.

[101] Rojas LBA, Gomes MB. Metformin: an old but still the best treatment for type 2 diabetes. Diabetol Metab Syndr. 2013 Feb;5(1):6.

[102] Cook MN, Girman CJ, Stein PP, Alexander CM. Initial monotherapy with either metformin or sulphonylureas often fails to achieve or maintain current glycaemic goals in patients with Type 2 diabetes in UK primary care. Diabet Med. 2007 Apr;24(4):350–8.

[103] Graham GG, Punt J, Arora M, Day RO, Doogue MP, Duong JK, et al. Clinical pharmacokinetics of metformin. Clin Pharmacokinet. 2011 Feb;50(2):81–98.

[104] Yoon H, Cho H-Y, Yoo H-D, Kim S-M, Lee Y-B. Influences of organic cation transporter polymorphisms on the population pharmacokinetics of metformin in healthy subjects. AAPS J. 2013 Apr;15(2):571–80.

[105] Menjivar M, Sánchez-Pozos K, Jaimes-Santoyo J, Monroy-Escutia J, Rivera-Santiago C, de Los Ángeles Granados-Silvestre M, et al. Pharmacogenetic Evaluation of Metformin and Sulphonylurea Response in Mexican Mestizos with Type 2 Diabetes. Curr Drug Metab. 2020;21(4):291–300.

[106] Raj GM, Mathaiyan J, Wyawahare M, Priyadarshini R. Lack of effect of the SLC47A1 and SLC47A2 gene polymorphisms on the glycemic response to metformin in type 2 diabetes mellitus patients. Drug Metab Pers Ther. 2018 Dec;33(4):175–85.

[107] Dujic T, Zhou K, Yee SW, van Leeuwen N, de Keyser CE, Javorský M,

et al. Variants in Pharmacokinetic Transporters and Glycemic Response to Metformin: A Metgen Meta-Analysis. Clin Pharmacol Ther. 2017 Jun;101(6): 763–72.

[108] Sola D, Rossi L, Schianca GPC, Maffioli P, Bigliocca M, Mella R, et al. Sulfonylureas and their use in clinical practice. Arch Med Sci. 2015 Aug;11(4): 840–8.

[109] Tahrani AA, Barnett AH, Bailey CJ. Pharmacology and therapeutic implications of current drugs for type 2 diabetes mellitus. Nat Rev Endocrinol. 2016 Oct;12(10):566–92.

[110] Le P, Chaitoff A, Misra-Hebert AD, Ye W, Herman WH, Rothberg MB. Use of Antihyperglycemic Medications in U.S. Adults: An Analysis of the National Health and Nutrition Examination Survey. Diabetes Care. 2020 Jun;43(6):1227–33.

[111] DeFronzo RA. Pharmacologic therapy for type 2 diabetes mellitus. Vol. 133, Annals of internal medicine. United States; 2000. p. 73–4.

[112] Seino S, Sugawara K, Yokoi N, Takahashi H. β-Cell signalling and insulin secretagogues: A path for improved diabetes therapy. Diabetes, Obes Metab. 2017;19(S1):22–9.

[113] Dunkley AJ, Fitzpatrick C, Gray LJ, Waheed G, Heller SR, Frier BM, et al. Incidence and severity of hypoglycaemia in type 2 diabetes by treatment regimen: A UK multisite 12-month prospective observational study. Diabetes Obes Metab. 2019 Jul;21(7): 1585–95.

[114] Zoungas S, Patel A, Chalmers J, de Galan BE, Li Q, Billot L, et al. Severe hypoglycemia and risks of vascular events and death. N Engl J Med. 2010 Oct;363(15):1410–8.

[115] Miller CD, Phillips LS, Ziemer DC, Gallina DL, Cook CB, El-Kebbi IM. Hypoglycemia in patients with type 2 diabetes mellitus. Arch Intern Med. 2001 Jul;161(13):1653–9.

[116] Risk of hypoglycaemia in types 1 and 2 diabetes: effects of treatment modalities and their duration. Diabetologia. 2007 Jun;50(6):1140–7.

[117] Aquilante CL. Sulfonylurea pharmacogenomics in Type 2 diabetes: the influence of drug target and diabetes risk polymorphisms. Expert Rev Cardiovasc Ther. 2010 Mar;8(3):359–72.

[118] Zhang H-F, Wang H-H, Gao N, Wei J-Y, Tian X, Zhao Y, et al. Physiological Content and Intrinsic Activities of 10 Cytochrome P450 Isoforms in Human Normal Liver Microsomes. J Pharmacol Exp Ther. 2016 Jul;358(1):83–93.

[119] Isvoran A, Louet M, Vladoiu DL, Craciun D, Loriot M-A, Villoutreix BO, et al. Pharmacogenomics of the cytochrome P450 2C family: impacts of amino acid variations on drug metabolism. Drug Discov Today. 2017 Feb;22(2):366–76.

[120] Daly AK, Rettie AE, Fowler DM, Miners JO. Pharmacogenomics of CYP2C9: Functional and Clinical Considerations. J Pers Med. 2017 Dec;8(1).

[121] Ragia G, Petridis I, Tavridou A, Christakidis D, Manolopoulos VG. Presence of CYP2C9*3 allele increases risk for hypoglycemia in Type 2 diabetic patients treated with sulfonylureas. Pharmacogenomics. 2009 Nov;10(11): 1781–7.

[122] Nasykhova YA, Tonyan ZN, Mikhailova AA, Danilova MM, Glotov AS. Pharmacogenetics of Type 2 Diabetes-Progress and Prospects. Int J Mol Sci. 2020 Sep;21(18).

[123] McTaggart JS, Clark RH, Ashcroft FM. The role of the KATP

channel in glucose homeostasis in health and disease: more than meets the islet. J Physiol. 2010 Sep;588(Pt 17):3201–9.

[124] Emdin CA, Klarin D, Natarajan P, Florez JC, Kathiresan S, Khera A V. Genetic Variation at the Sulfonylurea Receptor, Type 2 Diabetes, and Coronary Heart Disease. Diabetes. 2017 Aug;66(8):2310–5.

[125] Cordiner RLM, Pearson ER. Reflections on the sulphonylurea story: A drug class at risk of extinction or a drug class worth reviving? Diabetes Obes Metab. 2019 Apr;21(4):761–71.

[126] Florez JC, Jablonski KA, Kahn SE, Franks PW, Dabelea D, Hamman RF, et al. Type 2 diabetes-associated missense polymorphisms KCNJ11 E23K and ABCC8 A1369S influence progression to diabetes and response to interventions in the Diabetes Prevention Program. Diabetes. 2007 Feb;56(2): 531–6.

[127] Hansen T, Echwald SM, Hansen L, Møller AM, Almind K, Clausen JO, et al. Decreased tolbutamide-stimulated insulin secretion in healthy subjects with sequence variants in the high-affinity sulfonylurea receptor gene. Diabetes. 1998 Apr;47(4):598–605.

[128] Rissanen J, Markkanen A, Kärkkäinen P, Pihlajamäki J, Kekäläinen P, Mykkänen L, et al. Sulfonylurea receptor 1 gene variants are associated with gestational diabetes and type 2 diabetes but not with altered secretion of insulin. Diabetes Care. 2000 Jan;23(1):70–3.

[129] Quan Y, Barszczyk A, Feng Z, Sun H. Current understanding of K ATP channels in neonatal diseases: focus on insulin secretion disorders. Acta Pharmacol Sin. 2011 Jun;32(6):765–80.

[130] Villareal DT, Koster JC, Robertson H, Akrouh A, Miyake K, Bell GI, et al. Kir6.2 variant E23K increases ATP-sensitive K+ channel activity and is associated with impaired insulin release and enhanced insulin sensitivity in adults with normal glucose tolerance. Diabetes. 2009 Aug;58(8): 1869–78.

[131] Florez JC, Burtt N, de Bakker PIW, Almgren P, Tuomi T, Holmkvist J, et al. Haplotype structure and genotype-phenotype correlations of the sulfonylurea receptor and the islet ATP-sensitive potassium channel gene region. Diabetes. 2004 May;53(5): 1360–8.

[132] Sesti G, Laratta E, Cardellini M, Andreozzi F, Del Guerra S, Irace C, et al. The E23K variant of KCNJ11 encoding the pancreatic beta-cell adenosine 5'-triphosphate-sensitive potassium channel subunit Kir6.2 is associated with an increased risk of secondary failure to sulfonylurea in patients with type 2 diabetes. J Clin Endocrinol Metab. 2006 Jun;91(6):2334–9.

[133] Holstein A, Hahn M, Stumvoll M, Kovacs P. The E23K variant of KCNJ11 and the risk for severe sulfonylurea-induced hypoglycemia in patients with type 2 diabetes. Horm Metab Res = Horm und Stoffwechselforsch = Horm Metab. 2009 May;41(5):387–90.

[134] Haghvirdizadeh P, Mohamed Z, Abdullah NA, Haghvirdizadeh P, Haerian MS, Haerian BS. KCNJ11: Genetic Polymorphisms and Risk of Diabetes Mellitus. J Diabetes Res. 2015; 2015:908152.

[135] Ohshige T, Tanaka Y, Araki S, Babazono T, Toyoda M, Umezono T, et al. A single nucleotide polymorphism in KCNQ1 is associated with susceptibility to diabetic nephropathy in japanese subjects with type 2 diabetes. Diabetes Care. 2010 Apr;33(4):842–6.

[136] Barhanin J, Lesage F, Guillemare E, Fink M, Lazdunski M, Romey G. K(V) LQT1 and lsK (minK) proteins associate

to form the I(Ks) cardiac potassium current. Nature. 1996 Nov;384(6604): 78–80.

[137] Ullrich S, Su J, Ranta F, Wittekindt OH, Ris F, Rösler M, et al. Effects of I(Ks) channel inhibitors in insulin-secreting INS-1 cells. Pflugers Arch. 2005 Dec;451(3):428–36.

[138] Grant SFA, Thorleifsson G, Reynisdottir I, Benediktsson R, Manolescu A, Sainz J, et al. Variant of transcription factor 7-like 2 (TCF7L2) gene confers risk of type 2 diabetes. Nat Genet. 2006 Mar;38(3):320–3.

[139] da Silva Xavier G, Loder MK, McDonald A, Tarasov AI, Carzaniga R, Kronenberger K, et al. TCF7L2 regulates late events in insulin secretion from pancreatic islet beta-cells. Diabetes. 2009 Apr;58(4):894–905.

[140] Zhou Y, Park S-Y, Su J, Bailey K, Ottosson-Laakso E, Shcherbina L, et al. TCF7L2 is a master regulator of insulin production and processing. Hum Mol Genet. 2014 Dec;23(24):6419–31.

[141] Dhawan D, Padh H. Genetic variations in TCF7L2 influence therapeutic response to sulfonylureas in Indian diabetics. Diabetes Res Clin Pract. 2016 Nov;121:35–40.

[142] Gunawardana SC, Rocheleau J V, Head WS, Piston DW. Mechanisms of time-dependent potentiation of insulin release: involvement of nitric oxide synthase. Diabetes. 2006 Apr;55(4): 1029–33.

[143] Schulz R, Rassaf T, Massion PB, Kelm M, Balligand J-L. Recent advances in the understanding of the role of nitric oxide in cardiovascular homeostasis. Pharmacol Ther. 2005;108(3):225–56.

[144] Treuer A V, Gonzalez DR. NOS1AP modulates intracellular Ca(2+) in cardiac myocytes and is up-regulated in dystrophic cardiomyopathy. Int J Physiol Pathophysiol Pharmacol. 2014;6 (1):37–46.

[145] Cho H-J, Lee S-Y, Kim Y-G, Oh S-Y, Kim J-W, Huh W, et al. Effect of genetic polymorphisms on the pharmacokinetics and efficacy of glimepiride in a Korean population. Clin Chim Acta. 2011 Sep;412(19–20): 1831–4.

[146] Sherifali D, Nerenberg K, Pullenayegum E, Cheng JE, Gerstein HC. The effect of oral antidiabetic agents on A1C levels: a systematic review and meta-analysis. Diabetes Care. 2010 Aug;33(8):1859–64.

[147] Kahn SE, Haffner SM, Heise MA, Herman WH, Holman RR, Jones NP, et al. Glycemic durability of rosiglitazone, metformin, or glyburide monotherapy. N Engl J Med. 2006 Dec; 355(23):2427–43.

[148] Bailey CJ. Safety of antidiabetes medications: An update. Clin Pharmacol Ther. 2015 Aug;98(2):185–95.

[149] Yki-Järvinen H. Thiazolidinediones. N Engl J Med. 2004 Sep;351(11):1106–18.

[150] Baldwin SJ, Clarke SE, Chenery RJ. Characterization of the cytochrome P450 enzymes involved in the in vitro metabolism of rosiglitazone. Br J Clin Pharmacol. 1999 Sep;48(3):424–32.

[151] Chang C, Pang KS, Swaan PW, Ekins S. Comparative pharmacophore modeling of organic anion transporting polypeptides: a meta-analysis of rat Oatp1a1 and human OATP1B1. J Pharmacol Exp Ther. 2005 Aug;314(2): 533–41.

[152] Aquilante CL, Bushman LR, Knutsen SD, Burt LE, Rome LC, Kosmiski LA. Influence of SLCO1B1 and CYP2C8 gene polymorphisms on rosiglitazone pharmacokinetics in

healthy volunteers. Hum Genomics. 2008 Sep;3(1):7–16.

[153] Lebovitz HE, Banerji MA. Insulin resistance and its treatment by thiazolidinediones. Recent Prog Horm Res. 2001;56:265–94.

[154] Olefsky JM, Saltiel AR. PPAR gamma and the treatment of insulin resistance. Trends Endocrinol Metab. 2000 Nov;11(9):362–8.

[155] Sears DD, Hsiao G, Hsiao A, Yu JG, Courtney CH, Ofrecio JM, et al. Mechanisms of human insulin resistance and thiazolidinedione-mediated insulin sensitization. Proc Natl Acad Sci U S A. 2009 Nov;106(44):18745–50.

[156] Sarhangi N, Sharifi F, Hashemian L, Hassani Doabsari M, Heshmatzad K, Rahbaran M, et al. PPARG (Pro12Ala) genetic variant and risk of T2DM: a systematic review and meta-analysis. Sci Rep. 2020 Jul;10(1):12764.

[157] Tamori Y, Masugi J, Nishino N, Kasuga M. Role of peroxisome proliferator-activated receptor-gamma in maintenance of the characteristics of mature 3T3-L1 adipocytes. Diabetes. 2002 Jul;51(7):2045–55.

[158] Vasilatou D, Papageorgiou SG, Dimitriadis G, Pappa V. Epigenetic alterations and microRNAs: new players in the pathogenesis of myelodysplastic syndromes. Epigenetics. 2013 Jun;8(6): 561–70.

[159] Green BD, Flatt PR, Bailey CJ. Dipeptidyl peptidase IV (DPP IV) inhibitors: A newly emerging drug class for the treatment of type 2 diabetes. Diabetes Vasc Dis Res. 2006 Dec;3(3): 159–65.

[160] Hopsu-Havu VK, Glenner GG. A new dipeptide naphthylamidase hydrolyzing glycyl-prolyl-beta-naphthylamide. Histochemie. 1966;7(3): 197–201.

[161] Jose T, Inzucchi SE. Cardiovascular effects of the DPP-4 inhibitors. Diabetes Vasc Dis Res. 2012 Apr;9(2):109–16.

[162] Brown DX, Evans M. Choosing between GLP-1 Receptor Agonists and DPP-4 Inhibitors: A Pharmacological Perspective. J Nutr Metab. 2012;2012: 381713.

[163] Röhrborn D, Wronkowitz N, Eckel J. DPP4 in Diabetes. Front Immunol. 2015;6:386.

[164] Krittanawong C, Xanthopoulos A, Kitai T, Branis N, Zhang H, Kukin M. DPP-4 inhibitors and heart failure: a potential role for pharmacogenomics. Heart Fail Rev. 2018 May;23(3):355–61.

[165] Neumiller JJ, White JRJ, Campbell RK. Sodium-glucose co-transport inhibitors: progress and therapeutic potential in type 2 diabetes mellitus. Drugs. 2010 Mar;70(4):377–85.

[166] Nair S, Wilding JPH. Sodium glucose cotransporter 2 inhibitors as a new treatment for diabetes mellitus. J Clin Endocrinol Metab. 2010 Jan;95(1): 34–42.

[167] Zimdahl H, Haupt A, Brendel M, Bour L, Machicao F, Salsali A, et al. Influence of common polymorphisms in the SLC5A2 gene on metabolic traits in subjects at increased risk of diabetes and on response to empagliflozin treatment in patients with diabetes. Pharmacogenet Genomics. 2017 Apr;27(4):135–42.

[168] Lauschke VM, Ingelman-Sundberg M. Prediction of drug response and adverse drug reactions: From twin studies to Next Generation Sequencing. Eur J Pharm Sci Off J Eur Fed Pharm Sci. 2019 Mar;130:65–77.

[169] Ingelman-Sundberg M, Gomez A. The past, present and future of pharmacoepigenomics. Pharmacogenomics. 2010 May;11(5): 625–7.

[170] Harvey ZH, Chen Y, Jarosz DF. Protein-Based Inheritance: Epigenetics beyond the Chromosome. Mol Cell. 2018 Jan;69(2):195–202.

[171] Delcuve GP, Rastegar M, Davie JR. Epigenetic control. J Cell Physiol. 2009 May;219(2):243–50.

[172] Diehl P, Fricke A, Sander L, Stamm J, Bassler N, Htun N, et al. Microparticles: major transport vehicles for distinct microRNAs in circulation. Cardiovasc Res. 2012 Mar;93(4):633–44.

[173] Sekar D, Venugopal B, Sekar P, Ramalingam K. Role of microRNA 21 in diabetes and associated/related diseases. Gene. 2016 May;582(1):14–8.

[174] Rottiers V, Näär AM. MicroRNAs in metabolism and metabolic disorders. Nat Rev Mol Cell Biol. 2012 Mar;13(4): 239–50.

[175] Fu X, Dong B, Tian Y, Lefebvre P, Meng Z, Wang X, et al. MicroRNA-26a regulates insulin sensitivity and metabolism of glucose and lipids. J Clin Invest. 2015 Jun;125(6):2497–509.

[176] Janssen HLA, Reesink HW, Lawitz EJ, Zeuzem S, Rodriguez-Torres M, Patel K, et al. Treatment of HCV infection by targeting microRNA. N Engl J Med. 2013 May;368(18):1685–94.

[177] Ingelman-Sundberg M, Sim SC. Pharmacogenetic biomarkers as tools for improved drug therapy; emphasis on the cytochrome P450 system. Biochem Biophys Res Commun. 2010 May;396 (1):90–4.

[178] Lauschke VM, Barragan I, Ingelman-Sundberg M. Pharmacoepigenetics and Toxicoepigenetics: Novel Mechanistic Insights and Therapeutic Opportunities. Annu Rev Pharmacol Toxicol. 2018 Jan; 58:161–85.

Chapter 4

Metabolism of Phytochemicals

Tanu Dixit, Akash Tiwari, Sneha Bose, Himani Kulkarni, Jitendra Suthar and Selvan Ravindran

Abstract

Several phytochemicals have been developed as medicinal compounds. Extensive research has recently been conducted on phytochemicals such as curcumin, resveratrol, catechin, gallic acid, humulone, quercetin, rutin, diosgenin, allicin, gingerenone-A, caffeic acid, ellagic acid, kaempferol, isorhamnetin, chlorogenic acid, and others. All of these phytochemicals are metabolized in the biological system. To study the metabolic pathways of phytochemicals, studies are done using both *in vitro* and *in vivo* techniques. Metabolism is critical in determining phytochemical bioavailability, pharmacokinetics, and effectiveness. Metabolism can occur in organs such as the intestine, liver, gut, and spleen. The metabolic process is aided by a variety of enzymes, including cytochrome P450 enzymes found in the organs. This study outlines a few phytochemicals metabolic pathways. Tannic acid, ellagic acid, curcumin, quercetin, and resveratrol are selected and explained as examples.

Keywords: metabolism, phytochemicals, biotransformation, natural products, metabolic pathways, medicinal compounds

1. Introduction

More phytochemicals are extensively researched in the past several years. Still, curiosity among researchers for medicinally important phytochemicals is increasing. Recently, during the outbreak of the coronavirus, several scientists around the world are in search of various modalities of treatment and one among them was through phytochemicals or naturally available compounds.

Formononetin, scutellarin, emodin, withanone, escin, quabin, tannic acid, genistein, and other naturally derived phytochemicals are being researched for their capacity to cure Middle East Respiratory Syndrome - Coronavirus (MERS-CoV), which causes Middle East respiratory syndrome. Pharmaceutical drugs developed based on the phytochemicals have been authorized by the Food and Drug Administration (FDA) for use in the treatment of different illnesses [1].

Phytochemicals derived from plants, marine-derived, and fungus are the source to discover drugs and prevent disease [2].

Several natural products exhibit antiviral effects against human CoVs, which will help to develop antiviral prophylactics. Phytochemicals such as dihydrotanshinone, quabin, and griffthsin suppress MERS-CoV by targeting the virus's S protein and preventing viral entrance [3–6]. Therefore, this chapter highlights few examples from the literature and the importance of metabolism study in drug discovery and development.

Before a pharmaceutical drug is approved by the FDA, its metabolites are thoroughly researched and described, as well as related *in vitro* and *in vivo* investigations [7–11].

Similar rigorous studies are essential for phytochemicals, nanomedicine [12–15], monoclonal antibodies [16], formulation materials, and other new forms of therapeutics.

Upon successful completion of pharmacological and toxicological studies, the desired phytochemicals can be scaled up using bioreactors with the aid of microorganisms [17] or a methodology can be developed to synthesize the compounds by biological methods [18].

2. Metabolism of tannic acid

Tannic acid metabolism in male wistar rats was investigated *in vivo*. Tannic acid solutions containing 1 gram of tannic acid in 10 mL of water were administered at a rate of 10 mL per kilogram of body weight. Tannic acid was also given orally at a dosage of 1 g per kilogram, and serum was collected at various time intervals. Similarly, urine and fecal samples were collected at different times.

The most abundant metabolites in blood samples were 4-O-methyl gallic acid (4-OMGA), pyrogallol, and resorcinol. The highest concentration of 4-O-methyl gallic acid (4-OMGA) was found 1.5 hours after injection. Similarly, the highest levels of pyrogallol and resorcinol were found at 4 and 17 hours, respectively.

Urine contains four distinct metabolites: 4-O-methyl gallic acid, gallic acid, resorcinol, and pyrogallol. The metabolite 4-O-methyl pyrogallol was not found in the feces. The presence of gallic acid in the liver, which is eliminated through urine, was confirmed by analysis of metabolites present in serum, urine, and fecal samples (**Figure 1**) [19].

Tannic acid and theaflavin-3-gallate, two natural polyphenols present in black tea, have been shown to inhibit SARS-CoV, with IC50 values of 3 and 7 micromolars, respectively. As a result, investigations on the metabolism of tannic acid and theoflavin-3-gallate are becoming increasingly essential [20].

Recent research suggests that theaflavin metabolites of microbial origin derived from black tea intake are the primary cause of its positive benefits. Microbial

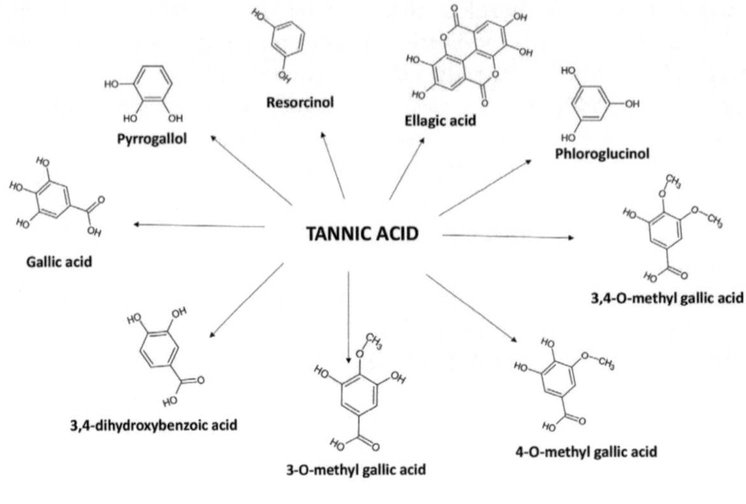

Figure 1.
Metabolic pathway of tannic acid in the rat [7].

biotransformation products 3.4-dihydroxybenzoic acid and phloroglucinol, as well as their corresponding sulfate and glucuronide conjugates, have been shown to lower pro-inflammatory chemokine levels, as well as molecules such as TNF-alpha, IL-6 in CD4L, oxidized LDL-challenged vascular endothelial cells, and sVCAM-1 [21].

In a reported study, healthy humans were ingested with 1 g of theoflavin extract and their urine and fecal samples were analyzed by high-resolution chromatography and mass spectrometry [22].

Theaflavins from black tea have low bioavailability, according to research. A sufficient amount of theaflavin enters the colon while traveling through the GI tract, where bacteria attack it, resulting in low-molecular-weight metabolites [23].

Additional metabolites for theoflavin have been found as 3-(4′-hydroxyphenyl) propionic acid and gallic acid. According to research, these intestinal metabolites act as agents against the progression of neurodegenerative disorders and have the ability to shield brain cells from oxidative stress. In human colon cancer cells, gallic acid inhibits cell proliferation and causes apoptosis.

3. Metabolism of polyphenols in tea

Many scientists are curious about the metabolism of green tea after it has been taken by humans. Human participants were given 500-mL bottles of green tea, and over 24 hours, urine and plasma samples were collected for the study. Green tea includes flavan-3-ols, (−)-epigallocatechin, (−)-epicatechin, (+)-gallocatechin, (−)-epigallocatechin-3-O-gallate (EGCG), and (−)-epicatechin-3-O-gallate (EgCG) [24].

The major epicatechin conjugates identified in the blood sample were (−)-epicatechin-3′-O-glucuronide, (−)-epicatechin-3′-O-sulfate, and 3′-O-methyl-(−)-epicatechin-O-sulfate.

4. Influence of chirality on metabolism

Another significant element of drug metabolism is chirality. Flavan-3-ols are chiral, and their potency and effect vary between enantiomers. According to research, (+)-catechin is more easily absorbed than (−)-catechin [25]. Similarly, comparative human studies about the bioavailability of (+)-catechin, (−)-catechin, (+)-epicatechin, and (−)-epicatechin reveals that (−) catechin is least bioavailable, followed by (+)-catechin, (+)-epicatechin, and (−)-epicatechin. These results were based on the analysis of urine and plasma samples from humans who consumed (−)-catechin, (+)-catechin, (+)-epicatechin, and (−)-epicatechin in equal quantity in a cocoa drink instead of green tea to avoid cross-contamination from flavan-3-ols present in green tea, which can alter the outcome of results [25, 26].

5. Metabolism of ellagic acid

Ellagitannins produce ellagic acid when exposed to basic or acidic environments. Ellagic acid was discovered to have antifungal, antiviral, anti-inflammatory, hepatoprotective, and cardioprotective effects [27].

Ellagic acid and ellagitannins are polyphenols found in berries, nuts, pomegranates, wines, and a range of medicinal herbs. Gut flora is necessary for the conversion of ellagitannins and ellagic acid to anticarcinogenic and anti-inflammatory metabolite urolithins (**Figure 2**).

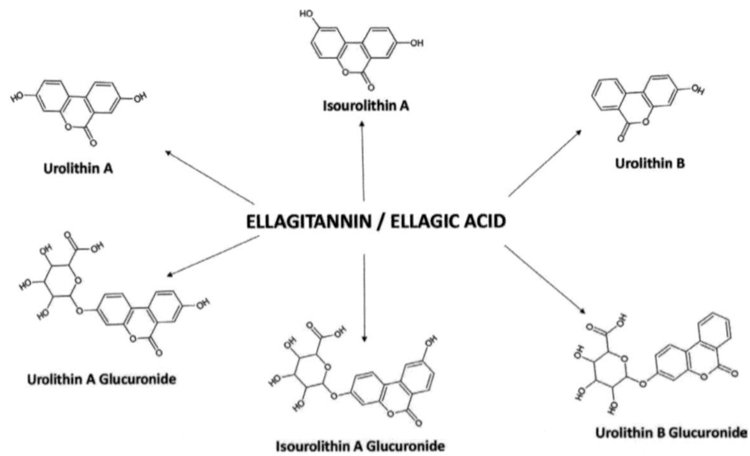

Figure 2.
Metabolism of ellagitannin/ellagic acid by human gut microbiota. Population genotypes have a significant influence on the metabolic pathway [28–30].

Ellagic acid and ellagitannins are classified under polyphenols and can be obtained from various natural sources such as pomegranates, nuts, wines, berries, and several medicinal plants. Gut bacteria are crucial in the conversion of both ellagitannins and ellagic acid to urolithin A and its glucuronide conjugate, urolithin B and its glucuronide conjugate, isourolithin A, and its glucuronide conjugate, which are anticarcinogenic and anti-inflammatory metabolites. These metabolites are highly bioavailable [27–29].

Recently, the metabolic conversion of ellagitannin/ellagic acid to urolithins was investigated in three distinct phenotypic populations. The criteria used to distinguish the population were age, body mass index, gender, and quantity of consumed ellagitannin. Subjects were given walnut and pomegranate extracts, and their urine profiles were analyzed carefully [30]. According to the study, population group A only displayed conjugates of urolithin A. Isourolithin A, urolithin A, and/or urolithin B were among the metabolites discovered in population group B. Metabolites were not identified in population group C. This study demonstrates that differences in human microbiota have a major influence in metabolite synthesis. The outcomes of the study were based on the excretion patterns of three different patient morphologies.

Ellagitannin is a phytochemical found in pomegranate juice, peel, and extracts. Microbial and human enzymes aid in the biotransformation of these phytochemicals. Pomegranate juice contains phytochemicals that have anti-inflammatory, anticancer, and anti-aging effects [31].

After injecting pomegranate juice into healthy volunteers, researchers discovered a maximum concentration of ellagic acid of about 0.06 micromolar in their blood circulation [32].

The gut microbiota of humans transforms ellagic acid into urolithins before its absorption by the intestinal cells. Ellagitannin metabolites were detected in human plasma, and some can be seen in urine for up to 48 hours [33]. One of the studies had confirmed that the plasma concentration of urolithin peaked at 18.6 micromolar in healthy volunteers after consumption of pomegranate juice on consecutive 5 days [34].

Similar studies were also performed using raspberry juice and blackberry juice. Urolithin metabolites were discovered and the urolithin excretion pattern was examined between patients with gut dysbiosis and healthy subjects [34, 35]. The primary metabolites observed throughout the metabolic process are isourolithin A, urolithin B, urolithin A glucuronide, isourolithin A glucuronide, and urolithin B glucuronide [31, 36].

6. Metabolism of curcumin

Curcumin is a major component of turmeric and is used as a remedy for many ailments. Curcumin is predominantly metabolized in the liver, along with gut and intestine. Reductase is responsible for the transformation of curcumin to its reduced form in enterocytes and hepatocytes. Curcumin's reductive phase-I metabolites are dihydrocurcumin, tetrahydrocurcumin, hexahydrocurcumin, and octahydrocurcumin which upon biotransformation produces glucuronide conjugates and sulfate conjugates as phase-II metabolites (**Figure 3**) [13].

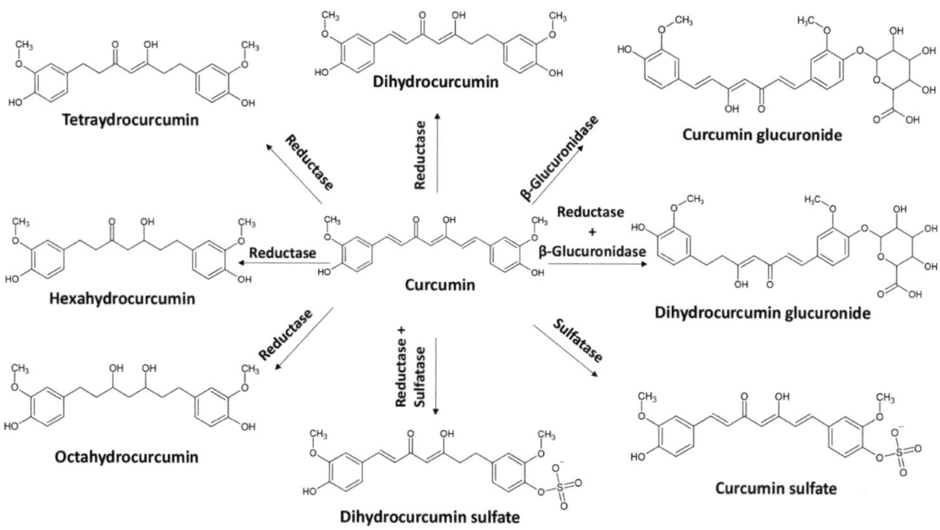

Figure 3.
Phase-I and phase-II metabolic pathway for curcumin.

7. Metabolism of quercetin and rutin

Quercetin is poorly absorbed in the stomach, but its primary site for absorption is the small intestine. Naturally, quercetin inbound to sugars and the sugar moiety is removed during absorption into the enterocytes by the lactase phloridzin hydrolase enzyme. After absorption quercetin is biotransformed to glucuronide conjugate through UDP-glucuronosyl transferases (UGTs), sulfate conjugates by sulfotransferases, and methylation through catechol-O-methyl transferase [37]. Hepatic and intestinal cells play a key role in metabolism (**Figure 4**).

A similar mechanism occurs in the gut where quercetin glucosides are absorbed and deglycosylated to quercetin aglycone with the assistance of enzymes present in the gut microbiota.

Rutin, consisting of quercetin moiety, is unabsorbed in the intestine but undergoes deglycosylation by β-glucosidases and α-rhamnosidases by the gut microbiota [38] followed by catabolic reactions to results in low-molecular-weight phenolic species (**Figure 5**).

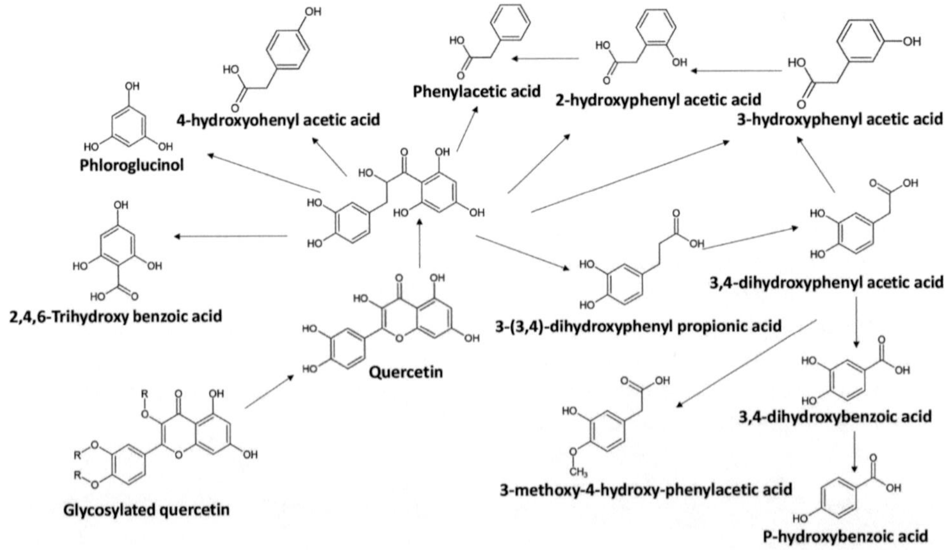

Figure 4.
Metabolic pathway for quercetin in gut.

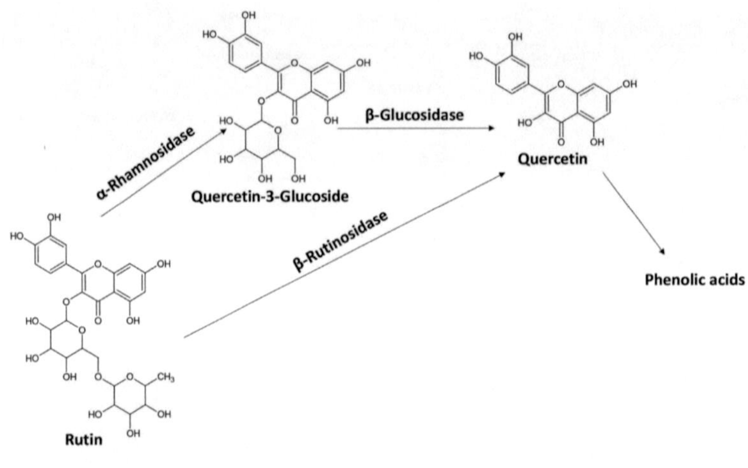

Figure 5.
Metabolic pathway of rutin by gut microbiota.

Author details

Tanu Dixit, Akash Tiwari, Sneha Bose, Himani Kulkarni, Jitendra Suthar and Selvan Ravindran*
Symbiosis School of Biological Sciences, Faculty of Health Sciences, Symbiosis International (Deemed) University, Pune, India

*Address all correspondence to: selvan_ravindran@yahoo.com; selvan.ravindran@ssbs.edu.in

References

[1] Patridge E, Gareiss P, Kinch MS, Hoyer D. An analysis of FDA approved drugs: Natural products and their derivatives. Drug Discovery Today. 2016;**21**:204-207. DOI: 10.1016/j.drudis.2015.01.009

[2] Wang D, Huang J, Yeung AWK, Tzvetkov NT, Horbańczuk JO, Willschke H, et al. The significance of natural product derivatives and traditional medicine for COVID-19. Processes. 2020;**8**:937. DOI: 10.3390/pr8080937

[3] Kim JY, Kim Y, Park SJ, Kim IK, Choi YK, Kim SH. Safe, high-throughput screening of natural compounds of MERS-CoV entry inhibitors using a pseudovirus expressing MERS-CoV spike protein. International Journal of Antimicrobial Agents. 2018;**52**:730-732. DOI: 10.1016/j.ijantimicag.2018.05.003

[4] Ko M, Chang SY, Byun SY, Choi I, d'Alexandry d'Orengiani ALPH, Shum D, et al. Screening of FDA-approved drugs using a MERS-CoV clinical isolate from South Korea identifies potential therapeutic options for COVID-19. bioRxiv. 2020:2020.02.25.965582. DOI: 10.1101/2020.02.25.965582

[5] Millet JK, Séron K, Labitt RN, Danneels A, Palmer KE, Whittaker GR, et al. Middle East respiratory syndrome coronavirus infection is inhibited by griffithsin. Antiviral Research. 2016;**133**:1-8. DOI: 10.1016/j.antiviral.2016.07.011

[6] Chen CN, Lin CPC, Huang KK, Chen WC, Hsieh HP, Liang PH, et al. Tannic acid and theaflavin-3-gallate are found to inhibit SARS-CoV by targeting 3CLPro and block the function of 3CLPro. Inhibition of SARS-CoV 3C-like protease activity by theaflavin–3,3′–digallate (TF3). Evidence-based Complementary and Alternative Medicine. 2005;**2**(2):209-215. DOI: 10.1093/ecam/neh081

[7] Ravindran S, Gorti SK, Basu S, Surve P, Honrao P. Differences and similarities in the metabolism of glyburide for various species: An analysis by LC-DAD-Q-TRAP-MS/MS. Journal of Analytical & Bioanalytical Techniques. 2013;**4**:164

[8] Ravindran S, HonRao C, Sahu R, Basu S, Basit A, Bharathi R, et al. Determining quantity of metabolites without synthetic standards: An approach using LC-PDA-MS. International Journal of Chemical and Analytical Science. 2011;**2**(10):1219-1221

[9] Khambadkar R, Ravindran S, Chahar DS, Utekar S, Tambe A. Qualitative and quantitative analysis of resveratrol and oxyresveratrol by liquid chromatography. Current Metabolomics and Systems Biology. Formerly Current Metabolomics. 2020;**7**(1):24-31

[10] Ravindran S, Zharikova OL, Hill RA, Nanovskaya TN, Hankins GD, Ahmed MS. Identification of glyburide metabolites formed by hepatic and placental microsomes of humans and baboons. Biochemical Pharmacology. 2006;**72**(12):1730-1737

[11] Ravindran S, Rokade R, Suthar J, Singh P, Deshpande P, Khambadkar R, et al. In vitro biotransformation in drug discovery. Concepts to Market. 2018;**1**:1-3

[12] Ravindran S, Suthar JK, Rokade R, Deshpande P, Singh P, Pratinidhi A, et al. Pharmacokinetics, metabolism, distribution and permeability of nanomedicine. Current Drug Metabolism. 2018;**19**(4):327-334

[13] Ravindran S, Tambe AJ, Suthar JK, Chahar DS, Fernandes JM, Desai V.

Nanomedicine: Bioavailability, biotransformation and biokinetics. Current Drug Metabolism. 2019;**20**(7): 542-555

[14] Suthar JK, Rokade R, Pratinidi A, Kambadkar R, Ravindran S. Purification of nanoparticles by liquid chromatography for biomedical and engineering applications. American Journal of Analytical Chemistry. 2017;**8**(10):617-624

[15] Shirolkar MM, Athavale R, Ravindran S, Rale V, Kulkarni A, Deokar R. Antibiotics functionalization intervened morphological, chemical and electronic modifications in chitosan nanoparticles. Nano-Structures & Nano-Objects. 2021;**25**:100657

[16] Chahar DS, Ravindran S, Pisal SS. Monoclonal antibody purification and its progression to commercial scale. Biologicals. 2020;**63**:1-3

[17] Ravindran S, Singh P, Nene S, Rale V, Mhetras N, Vaidya A. Microbioreactors and perfusion bioreactors for microbial and mammalian cell culture. Biotechnology and Bioengineering. 2019:1-13. DOI: http://dx.doi.org/10.5772/intechopen.83825

[18] Rokade R, Ravindran S, Singh P, Suthar JK. Microbial biotransformation for the production of steroid medicament. Secondary Metabolites - Sources and Applications. 2018:115-124

[19] Nakamura Y, Tsuji S, Tonogai Y. Method for Analysis of tannic acid and its metabolites in biological samples: Application to tannic acid metabolism in the rat. Journal of Agricultural and Food Chemistry. 2003;**51**:331-339

[20] Chen CN, Lin CPC, Huang KK, Chen WC, Hsieh HP, Liang PH, et al. Inhibition of SARS-CoV 3C-like protease activity by theaflavin–3,3′–digallate (TF3). Evidence-based Complementary and Alternative Medicine. 2005;**2**(2):209-215. DOI: 10.1093/ecam/neh081

[21] Amin HP, Czank C, Raheem S, Zhang Q, Botting NP, Cassidy A, et al. Anthocyanins and their physiologically relevant metabolites alter the expression of IL-6 and VCAM-1 in CD40L and oxidised LDL. Molecular Nutrition & Food Research. 2015;**50**(6):1095-1106

[22] Pereira-Caro G, Moreno-Rojas JM, Brindani N, Del-Rio D, Lean MEJ, Hata Y, et al. Bioavailability of black tea theaflavins: Absorption, metabolism and colonic catabolism. Journal of Agricultural and Food Chemistry. 2017;**65**(26):5365-5374

[23] Amin HP, Czank C, Raheem S, Zhang Q, Botting NP, Cassidy A, et al. Anthocyanins and their physiologically relevant metabolites alter the expression of IL-6 and VCAM-1 in CD40L and oxidized LDL challenged vascular endothelial cells. Molecular Nutrition & Food Research. 2015;**59**:1096-1106

[24] Stalmach A, Troufflard S, Serafini M, Crozier A. Absorption, metabolism and excretion of Choladi green tea flavan-3-ols by humans. Molecular Nutrition & Food Research. 2009;**53**:S44-S53

[25] Donovan JL, Crespy V, Oliveira M, Cooper KA, Gibson BB, Williamson G. (+)-Catechin is more bioavailable than (−)-catechin: Relevance to the bioavailability of catechin from cocoa. Free Radical Research. 2006;**40**:1029-1034

[26] Ottaviani JI, Momma TY, Heiss C, Kwik-Uribe C, Schroeter H, Keen CL. The stereochemical configuration of flavanols influences the level and metabolism of flavanols in humans and their biological activity in vivo. Free Radical Biology & Medicine. 2011;**50**:237-244

[27] Evtyugin DE, Magina S. Recent advances in the production and

applications of ellagic acid and its derivatives. A review. Molecules. 2020;**25**(12):2745

[28] Larrosa M, García-Conesa MT, Espín JC, Tomas-Barberan FA. Ellagitannins, ellagic acid and vascular health. Molecular Aspects of Medicine. 2010;**31**:513-539

[29] Espín JC, Larrosa M, García-Conesa MT, Tomas-Barberan FA. Biological significance of urolithins, the gut microbial ellagic acid derived metabolites: The evidence so far. Evidence-based Complementary and Alternative Medicine. 2013:1-15. DOI: 10.1155/2013/270418

[30] Seeram NP, Henning SM, Zhang Y, Suchard M, Li Z, Heber D. Pomegranate juice ellagitannin metabolites are present in human plasma and some persist in urine for up to 48 h. The Journal of Nutrition. 2006;**136**: 2481-2485

[31] Tomás-Barberán FA, García-Villalba R, González-Sarrías A, Selma MV, Espín JC. Ellagic acid metabolism by human gut microbiota: Consistent observation of three urolithin phenotypes in intervention trials, independent of food source, age, and health status. Journal of Agricultural and Food Chemistry. 2014;**62**(28):6535-6538. DOI: 10.1021/jf5024615

[32] Wu S, Tian L. Diverse phytochemicals and bioactivities in the ancient fruit and modern functional food pomegranate (*Punica granatum*). Molecules. 2017;**22**:1606. DOI: 10.3390/molecules22101606

[33] Seeram NP, Henning SM, Zhang Y, Suchard M, Li Z, Heber D. Pomegranate juice ellagitannin metabolites are present in human plasma and some persist in urine for up to 48 hours. The Journal of Nutrition. 2006;**136**: 2481-2485

[34] Cerdá B, Espín JC, Parra S, Martínez P, Tomás-Barberán FA. The potent in vitro antioxidant ellagitannins from pomegranate juice are metabolised into bioavailable but poor antioxidant hydroxy-6H-dibenzopyran-6-one derivatives by the colonic microflora of healthy humans. European Journal of Nutrition. 2004;**43**:205-220

[35] González-Barrio R, Borges G, Mullen W, Crozier A. Bioavailability of anthocyanins and ellagitannins following consumption of raspberries by healthy humans and subjects with an ileostomy. Journal of Agricultural and Food Chemistry. 2010;**58**:3933-3939

[36] García-Muñoz C, Hernández L, Pérez A, Vaillant F. Diversity of urinary excretion patterns of the main ellagitannins' colonic metabolites after ingestion of tropical highland blackberry (*Rubus adenotrichus*) juice. Food Research International. 2014;**55**: 161-169

[37] Almeida AF, Borge GIA, Piskula M, Tudose A, Tudoreanu L, Valentova K, et al. Bioavailability of quercetin in humans with a focus on interindividual variation. Comprehensive Reviews in Food Science and Food Safety. 2018;**17**: 714-731

[38] Riva A, Kolimar D, Splitter A, Wisgrill L, Herbold CW, Abranko L, et al. Conversion of Rutin, a prevalent dietary flavanol, by the human gut microbiota. Frontiers in Microbiology. 2020;**11**:1-11

Chapter 5

In vitro Metabolic Stability of Drugs and Applications of LC-MS in Metabolite Profiling

Marothu Vamsi Krishna, Kantamaneni Padmalatha and Gorrepati Madhavi

Abstract

Metabolic stability of a compound is an important factor to be considered during the early stages of drug discovery. If the compound has poor metabolic stability, it never becomes a drug even though it has promising pharmacological characteristics. For example, a drug is quickly metabolized in the body; it does not have sufficient *in vivo* exposure levels and leads to the production of toxic, non-active or active metabolites. A drug is slowly metabolized in the body it could remain longer periods in the body and lead to unwanted adverse reactions, toxicity or may cause drug interactions. Metabolic stability assay is performed to understand the susceptibility of the compound to undergo biotransformation in the body. Intrinsic clearance of the compound is measured by metabolic stability assays. Different *in vitro* test systems including liver microsomes, hepatocytes, S9 fractions, cytosol, recombinant expressed enzymes, and cell lines are used to investigate the metabolic stability of drugs. Metabolite profiling is a vital part of the drug discovery process and LC–MS plays a vital role. The development of high-resolution (HR) MS technologies with improved mass accuracy, in conjunction with novel data processing techniques, has significantly improved the metabolite detection and identification process. HR-MS based data acquisition (ion intensity-dependent acquisition, accurate-mass inclusion list-dependent acquisition, isotope pattern-dependent acquisition, pseudo neutral loss-dependent acquisition, and mass defect-dependent acquisition) and data mining techniques (extracted ion chromatogram, product ion filter, mass defect filter, isotope pattern filter, neutral loss filter, background subtraction, and control sample comparison) facilitate the drug metabolite identification process.

Keywords: metabolic stability, *in vitro* test systems, LC–MS, data acquisition and data mining techniques

1. Introduction

Drug metabolism is a process by which xenobiotics such as drugs are easily removed from the body by converting them into more polar derivatives and pharmacologically inactive. Nevertheless, sometimes metabolism makes the compound less soluble, toxic or pharmacologically active. Therefore, information on the metabolism of new drug candidate is important to know the possible toxicity and to circumvent failures in drug development. Bioavailability, half-life and clearance of a drug molecule are dependent on the rate of drug metabolism; these parameters define the dose and dosing frequency. A drug is difficult to develop, or market if the dose or dosing frequency is too high.

Drug metabolic reactions are two types, phase I and phase II biotransformation reactions. Hydrolysis, reduction, and oxidation are the phase I reactions catalyzed by cytochrome P450 (CYP) and flavin-containing monooxygenases (FMO). Phase II reactions are also called conjugation reactions in which metabolites produced in the phase I reactions may undergo glucuronide conjugation, glutathione conjugation, sulfoconjugation, amino acid conjugation, acetylation, and methylation. These reactions are catalyzed by enzymes like Uridine 5′-diphospho (UDP)-glucuronyl transferases (UGTs) or sulfotransferases (SULTs), glutathione *S*– transferases (GSTs), *N*–acetyltransferases (NATs), and methyltransferases [1–5]. *In vivo* pharmacokinetics are predicted by using *in vitro* metabolic stability studies in the early stages of drug discovery and development. Metabolic profile evaluation is also an important issue in this field [6–8].

Susceptibility of a chemical compound to biotransformation is known as metabolic stability and is articulated as intrinsic clearance (CL_{int}) and *in vitro* half-life ($t_{1/2}$). Intrinsic clearance (CL_{int}) is the ability of the liver to remove or metabolize the drug in the absence of flow restrictions and drug binding to cells, or proteins in the blood. $t_{1/2}$ is defined as the time required for 50% elimination of the parent compound. Different models are used to predict additional indices like hepatic clearance (CL_H), *in vivo* $t_{1/2}$, and bioavailability. Hepatic clearance (CL_H) is the most important parameter during drug development because most drugs are metabolized in the liver tissue [2, 9–13].

Metabolic stability of new drug molecule is assessed by *in vitro* techniques and then scaled to *in vivo* using scaling factors. When metabolic stability is performed with liver microsomes, *in vitro* half-life ($t_{1/2}$) can be determined from the slope of the linear regression of the percentage of drug remaining against time. Microsomal intrinsic clearance ($CL_{int,\ micr}$) can be determined using the equation $\ln 2/t_{1/2} \times$ [volume of incubation medium (μL)/microsomal protein in incubation (mg)] and the expressed units are μL min^{-1} mg^{-1}. *In vivo* intrinsic(hepatic)clearance is estimated from liver microsomal data using the equation $CL_{int} = CL_{int,micr} \times$ (mg microsome g^{-1} liver) × [liver mass (g)/body mass (kg)] and is expressed in the units of mL min^{-1} kg^{-1}. Scaling factors: 45 mg of microsomal protein per gram of liver tissue (humans, mice, rats, dogs, monkeys/value is applied to all species) and 26 g, 32 g, 30 g, 40 g and 87 g of liver tissue per kilogram of body weight is used for humans, monkeys, dogs, rats, and mice, respectively [2, 14–21].

McNaney *et al.* classified compounds based on their CL_{int} values, compounds with CL_{int} value above 15 mL min^{-1} kg^{-1} are called low clearance compounds, compounds with CL_{int} value between 15 and 45 mL min^{-1} kg^{-1} are called intermediate clearance compounds and compounds with CL_{int} values above 45 mL min^{-1} kg^{-1} are called as high clearance compounds [12]. High CL_{int} and low *in vitro* $t_{1/2}$ values indicate that the compound is rapidly metabolized and *in vivo* bioavailability of compound will be low. Hence, *in vitro* $t_{1/2}$ values can be used for the classification of compounds; for example in the case of human CYP3A4 supersomes, compounds with *in vitro* $t_{1/2}$value less than 10 min are classified as short *in vitro* $t_{1/2}$ compounds, compounds with *in vitro* $t_{1/2}$ value between 10 to 30 min are classified as moderate $t_{1/2}$ agents and long $t_{1/2}$ compounds are the compounds with *in vitro* $t_{1/2}$ value greater than 30 min [22].

A new chemical entity, which is suitable as a drug candidate must maintain adequate concentration at the site of action and could be slowly removed from the body to make sure of its action. High metabolic stability, high clearance values, and active or toxic metabolites formation are the biggest challenges during the drug discovery and development stages [23]. Compounds which have high clearance values are quickly removed from the body and show short duration of action. Conversely, compounds with low clearance values will show prolonged half-life and long duration of action, and so dosing will be reduced [24–28]. An important step in the drug discovery process is the identification of compounds with suitable metabolic profiles [29–31]; hence, the study of the chemical structure of molecule and identification of "soft spots" liable for biotransformation is required. Metabolic properties of the compound are improved by modification, or removal of the soft spots in the molecule [32, 33].

It is very important to carry out the metabolic stability of new molecules during the early stages of drug discovery to learn the metabolic characteristics. Even though some molecules pass in the *in vitro* level tests by showing promising results, they fail in the pharmacological and toxicological results at the *in vivo* level [24].

In vivo animal studies give important information regarding the metabolism of new chemical compounds, but these are costly, require more time, and are not suitable to test a large number of compounds. Hence, *in vitro* tests are used initially for the selection of compounds, and then a suitable animal model will be used in the drug development stages to determine the metabolic characteristics of selected compounds [23, 34–36]. During the drug discovery process, performance of metabolic stability by *in vitro* models is preferable compared with the animal models because the number of compounds to be tested is large and the amount of compound available for testing is small. Data from the *in vitro* metabolic studies will be useful for the targeted synthesis of compounds with required metabolic profiles and hence reduces the cost and time [2, 7, 37, 38].

2. *In vitro* test systems to conduct metabolic stability

Metabolic stability study can be conducted by incubating the test compound with the appropriate metabolic model (e.g., liver microsomes, hepatocytes, S9 fractions) and analysis of incubation mixture by suitable analytical techniques like LC–MS/MS [39–41].

Microsomes and hepatocytes are the commonly used *in vitro* systems to conduct metabolic stability. Other systems used are S9 fractions, cytosol, recombinant expressed enzymes, and cell lines.

2.1 Liver microsomes

Microsomes obtained from different species (e.g., human liver microsomes, HLM; rat liver microsomes, RLM; mouse liver microsomes, MLM; dog liver microsomes, DLM, or monkey liver microsomes, MnLM) are used in the metabolic stability studies [42]. The most popular *in vitro* model is human liver microsomes. Alternatively, MLM is a good preliminary tool that the results obtained correlate well with the results obtained with HLM [43, 44]. Liver microsomes are subcellular fractions derived from the smooth endoplasmic reticulum of liver cells. Homogenization of the liver and then differential centrifugation is performed to prepare the liver microsomes [9, 45]. Phase I oxidation is evaluated by the addition of a cofactor like nicotinamide adenine dinucleotide phosphate (NADP). Glucuronidation is also studied by liver microsomes with the addition of uridine diphosphate glucuronic acid (UDPGA). Various metabolizing enzymes like cytochrome P450s (CYP), flavin monooxygenases (FMO), epoxide hydrolase and carboxyl esterases, and UDP glucuronyl transferases are present in the HLM preparation. Hence, they are commonly used to study the metabolic fate of drugs [46].

Metabolic stability assays are generally performed by incubating the compound with liver microsomes and depletion of a drug during incubation is measured by HPLC or LC–MS. In the metabolic stability assay, the incubation mixture consists of a test compound (which is dissolved in potassium phosphate buffer, if not soluble in phosphate buffer dissolved in acetonitrile, methanol, or DMSO and the final organic solvent concentration in the assay should always be $\leq$1% for acetonitrile and methanol or $\leq$ 0.2% for DMSO), NADPH (reduced form of nicotinamide adenine dinucleotide phosphate) or NADPH regenerating system, potassium phosphate buffer and liver microsomes. Protein concentration usually does not exceed 2 mg/mL to prevent too much nonspecific binding. In the first step, the mixture containing the test compound, buffer, and microsomes is pre-incubated at 37°C for 15 minutes before the addition of NADPH. The obtained mixture is incubated at 37°C for several time intervals (*e.g.*, 15, 30, and 60 min). Incubation time is generally not more than 60 min for optimal conditions for enzymatic activity. At the predetermined time points, the reaction is quenched by the addition of ice-cold acetonitrile or methanol. The samples are vortexed and centrifuged; the supernatant is collected and analyzed by HPLC or LC–MS/MS. In the case of control samples, NADPH is replaced by potassium phosphate buffer [2, 24, 47–52].

The extent of metabolism (as substrate depletion) is calculated by using the following Equation [53].

$$\text{rate of depletion}\,(\text{pmol}/\text{min}/\text{mg}) = \frac{(\Delta C \times 1000)}{(B \times T)} \tag{1}$$

where ΔC = [concentration (or peak area) at 0 min] – [concentration (or peak area) at time T (nmol/mL or μM],

B is the microsome protein concentration (mg/mL),

T is the incubation time (min).

and 1000 is the conversion factor from nmol to pmol.

2.2 Hepatocytes

Phase I and Phase II drug metabolism is studied by using hepatocytes [9], which shows the heterogeneity of CYP expression in the human liver [54]. The metabolic profile of the number of drugs analyzed by cultured hepatocytes [55, 56] and suspensions of primary hepatocytes, and shown good *in vitro– in vivo* correlation [57–59]. A decrease in CYP expression is observed with cultured hepatocytes and thereby loss of liver specific functions. Phase I and Phase II enzyme activity is retained with cryopreserved hepatocytes. The disadvantage of hepatocytes may be an inter-individual variation that can be overcome by using mixtures of hepatocytes from different donors. HepatoPac is the new strategy used to create stable *in vitro* liver models that enable long-term hepatic metabolism and toxicity studies. It is a micropatterned hepatocyte-fibroblast co-culture system that can be used for continuous incubation of up to 7 days [2, 24, 28, 38, 60, 61].

The general procedure for a metabolic stability study is to prepare a hepatocyte suspension containing 10^6cells/mL and incubate for 10 min (37°C, 5% CO_2). Test compound solution is added to the cells and again incubated. At the predetermined time points (e.g., 15, 30, 60, and 90 min) reactions are stopped by the addition of ice-cold methanol or acetonitrile. Control samples are also prepared without hepatocytes. Supernatants are collected and analyzed for parent molecule and its metabolites by HPLC or LC–MS [43, 44, 60, 62–65].

2.3 Recombinant expressed enzymes

Recombinant expressed enzymes are the sources of specific P450 isoenzymes. The advantages are simplicity of the method and a single enzyme can be used for the study. In cases of low metabolism, recombinant enzymes can be used at high concentrations to increase metabolic activity for use in metabolic stability screening and in inhibitory potential evaluation. Recombinant enzymes can also be used in the confirmation of reaction phenotyping studies. Conversely, the absence of the remaining phase I and phase II enzymes can be considered as a disadvantage of this type of system [2, 66].

The assay procedure consists of a test compound solution, recombinant P450 isoenzyme, potassium phosphate buffer, and magnesium chloride. The mixture is pre-incubated for 15 min at 37°C and then the metabolic reaction is started by the addition of NADPH. The incubation is continued for different time points. The reaction is ended at each timepoint by the addition of ice cold acetonitrile or methanol and centrifuge the samples. Supernatants are collected and analyzed by HPLC or LC–MS [67, 68].

2.4 Cytosol

Cytosolic fraction is an *in vitro* model that has not been used commonly for biotransformation studies. The cytosol is produced by differential centrifugation of whole liver homogenate. Soluble enzymes of phase II, such as N-acetyltransferases (NAT), sulfotransferases (SULT), glutathione S-transferase (GST), carboxylesterase, diamine oxidase, soluble epoxide hydrolase, alcohol dehydrogenase, and xanthine oxidase are expressed in the cytosolic fraction, but the aforementioned initial three enzymes are expressed at higher concentration. This *in vitro* model requires cofactors like acetyl CoA (acetyl coenzyme A), acetyl CoA-regenerating system and dithiothreitol for NAT, 3′-phosphoadenosyl-5′-phosphosulfate (PAPS) for SULT, and glutathione for GST activity. The biotransformation by NAT, GST, or SULT can be studied separately or in combination depending on the cofactors added. The main disadvantage of this model is the lack of UGT and hence glucuronidation cannot be studied [69].

2.5 S9 fractions

S9 fraction preparations contain both cytosolic and microsomal fractions and as a result express a wide variety of metabolic enzymes-CYP, FMO, carboxylesterases, epoxide hydrolases, UGT, SULT, methyl transferases, acetyltransferases, GST, and others. This *in vitro* model can be used for metabolic, mutagenicity, and toxicity studies. The addition of co-factor is required for enzyme activity. The main advantage of S9 fraction over microsomes and cytosolic fraction is a more complete depiction of the metabolic profile due to the existence of phase I and phase II enzymes. In some cases, S9 fractions produce metabolites that are not formed by either microsomes or cytosol alone. However, the disadvantage of S9 fraction is overall lower enzyme activity compared with the microsomes and cytosol, thus it may leave some metabolites unnoticed [69, 70].

2.6 Cell lines

Cell lines are less popular than other described models due to de-differentiated cellular characteristics and absence of complete expression of all families of metabolic enzymes. The sources of cell lines are primary tumors of liver parenchyma. Currently, available cell lines include Hep G2, Hep3B, BC2, C3A, etc. Among them, the Hep G2 cell line is commonly used for biotransformation studies. Compared with the freshly isolated human hepatocytes, the metabolic activity of liver cell lines is generally low. Pretreatment of cell lines with various metabolic enzyme inducers partly reduces the problem of low activity. Even though, the induced activity is still below the enzymatic activity of freshly isolated human hepatocytes. An appropriate culture medium is required for the liver cell lines and the composition of the culture medium notably influences the metabolic activity. The described *in vitro* model is easy to culture and has steady enzyme concentration. Conversely, the lack or low expression of most important phase I and phase II drug metabolizing enzymes limits the application of this *in vitro* model. In addition, it is difficult to investigate individual enzymes due to their low expression level [70].

3. Metabolite profiling by LC-MS

Mass spectrometry plays an important role in the metabolite profiling of drugs during drug discovery and development. Quality and productivity of the metabolite identification process is improved by the availability of high-resolution (HR) MS instrumentation with superior accuracy and new data acquisition methods and data mining techniques. Hence, HPLC coupled with the high-resolution MS is the analytical tool of choice for metabolite profiling studies [71].

Drug metabolites can be categorized into expected metabolites and unexpected metabolites. Expected metabolites are those produced by common biotransformation reactions and are predictable, unexpected metabolites are those produced by uncommon reactions and are not easily predictable. Mass shift values from the parent drug can be used to calculate the molecular masses (*m/z* values) of expected metabolites. Acquisition of full-scan MS data using MS instrument, followed by extracted ion chromatography (EIC) of the ions can be used to accomplish the detection of expected metabolites by LC/MS [72, 73]. The most difficult task in drug metabolism studies is the detection and structural elucidation of very low levels of unexpected metabolites in the presence of endogenous interfering components [74–76].

Time-of-flight (TOF) and Fourier transform Orbitrap (Thermo Fisher Scientific) are the most commonly used high-resolution mass spectrometers in metabolite profiling of drugs. The principle involved in the TOF mass analyzers is ions of different *m/z* values having different velocities when accelerated by the same kinetic energy in the field-free flight tube. The time required for the ions to travel through the flight tube is proportional to the square root of their *m/z* values. The *m/z* value of each ion is determined by measuring the time taken for the ion to arrive at the detector. The resolution of the instrument is dependent on the capacity of the instrument to generate and maintain a focused ion beam through the ionization and acceleration region. The resolving power of the instrument is improved by utilizing reflectrons (reflecting ion mirrors), which decreases the spreading of kinetic energy among ions accelerated from the accelerator [77]. The ion saturation problem in the TOF instruments is effectively resolved by improvements in the ion detection technologies, for example, the use of segmented multichannel plates or analog-to-digital converters in place of time-to-digital converters. Modern TOF instruments offer good accuracy (~2–5 ppm), required resolution (~30,000) at full-width half maximum [FWHM]), and fast scan speed (20–50 spectra/second) [78, 79].

The Orbitrap mass analyzer consists of two electrodes, one is an outer barrel-like electrode and other is a coaxial inner spindle-like electrode. A static electric field is applied between the outer and inner electrodes. Around the central spindle electrode, ions are radially trapped, rotate about the inner electrode, and harmonically oscillated along the central electrode with a frequency characteristic to its mass to charge ratio (*m/z* value). An image current is produced on split outer electrodes due to the axial motion of the ions around the inner electrode. The mass spectrum is generated by fast Fourier transformation of the image current to convert the time-domain signal into a frequency, and then into an *m/z* spectrum [80, 81]. The Orbitrap MS offers good resolving power (~30,000–240,000) and mass accuracy (<3 ppm). The resolution of the Orbitrap instrument depends upon the scan speed; to achieve higher resolution, longer total cycle times are required. This is a limiting factor for the Orbitrap device to couple with the UPLC instruments in which peak width is only a few seconds. The most popular HRMS instrument configurations used for metabolite profiling are Q-TOF (quadrupole – time of flight) and LTQ (linear trap quadrupole) -Orbitrap, because of their high resolution and mass accuracy characteristics. A Q-TOF instrument consists of quadrupole, collision cell, and TOF mass analyzer. Q-TOF is obtained by switching the last quadrupole in the TQMS (triple quadrupole mass spectrometer) with TOF mass analyzer. It provides fast data acquisition, high sensitivity and resolution, and accurate mass on both MS and MS/MS modes, thus proven to be a powerful tool in metabolite profiling studies. LTQ (linear trap quadrupole) -Orbitrap is a hybrid mass spectrometer that combines a linear ion trap with Orbitrap MS. Accurate mass measurements are possible on multiple stages of fragmentation for structural elucidation of metabolites and MS^n (multi stage mass spectrometry) experiments can be performed simultaneously with ion trap detection while continuing mass measurements with Orbitrap. QExactive™ hybrid quadrupole - Orbitrap mass spectrometer combines quadrupole precursor ion selection with high resolution, accurate mass Orbitrap detection. It is compatible with fast chromatography techniques because of its high scan speed (~12 Hz) and spectral multiplexing capabilities; hence fit for high-throughput metabolite profiling. Current progress in HRMS leads to the development of various new data acquisition and data mining techniques for the rapid identification of drug metabolites.

3.1 Data acquisition methods for HRMS drug metabolite identification

Data acquisition methods used for metabolite identification include: ion intensity-dependent acquisition, accurate-mass inclusion list-dependent acquisition, isotope pattern-dependent acquisition, pseudo neutral loss-dependent acquisition, and mass defect-dependent acquisition [77].

3.1.1 Ion intensity-dependent acquisition

In this method, an ion intensity threshold is used to trigger the MS/MS acquisition of ions. Prior knowledge of the *m/z* values of the precursor ions is not required for this generic method. This method is very effective for *in vitro* metabolite profiling. Fifteen metabolites of nefazodone were identified from human liver microsomal incubations by applying intensity-dependent MS/MS acquisition of the three most intense ions from a single LC–MS/MS run [82]. This method is not suitable for complex biological samples because of matrix interferences. It is very difficult to acquire MS/MS spectra of trace level metabolites using this method because high-intensity endogenous ions are mainly selected for MS/MS or MS^n acquisition.

3.1.2 Accurate-mass inclusion list-dependent acquisition

This method uses a list of accurate masses of predicted or expected metabolites to trigger MS/MS acquisition of preset metabolite ions. Data analysis is performed by the software in real time to determine any mass in the list is detected in the full scan. If any ion is detected within a certain mass tolerance window and above a particular intensity threshold, the software will switch to MS/MS mode automatically and obtain the product ion (MS/MS) spectrum. This method increases the chance of getting MS/MS spectra for low level metabolites present in the complex biological samples. Moreover, in a single LC–MS/MS run both full-scan MS and MS/MS spectra of predicted metabolites will be obtained [83]. By using this approach and different post-acquisition data mining techniques, a total of 58*in vitro* metabolites of carvedilol were detected from human liver microsomal incubations [84].

On the other hand, preparation of an accurate mass inclusion list for every compound is time intensive and not suitable for high-throughput metabolite profiling during drug discovery. Besides, many of the major metabolites are generated by rearrangement, ring scission, or ring contraction and are hence difficult to predict.

3.1.3 Isotope pattern-dependent acquisition

Molecules containing elements like Cl and Br can be easily identified by their unique isotopic patterns in the mass spectra. Assume that during biotransformation these halogens remain intact and their unique isotopic pattern is used as a selective trigger for MS/MS acquisition of metabolite ions. It assists in the easy identification of metabolites and provides MS/MS spectra for structural analysis. The software is programmed such that any ion detected with a unique isotopic pattern (e.g., Cl-containing compounds: ion pairs with *m/z* difference of 1.99705 Da and an intensity ratio of 3:1; Br-containing compounds: ion pairs with *m/z* difference of 1.99795 Da and intensity ratio of 1:1) in the full scan MS would be automatically followed by an MS/MS experiment for rapid identification of metabolites. This approach has demonstrated to be very effective in metabolite profiling of a rat bile sample collected following a single oral dose (30 mg/kg) of a ^{14}C-bromine containing compound on a quadrupole time-of-flight mass spectrometer. Over 30 metabolites were detected with their MS/MS spectra automatically obtained in the same LC–MS/MS run [41]. Isotope pattern-dependent acquisition is also applicable to compounds containing synthetically incorporated isotopes (e.g.,^{2}H-, ^{13}C-,^{15}N-, ^{18}O-, etc.) or radiolabeled compound (^{14}C-) with a distinct ^{12}C/^{14}C isotopic pattern. Glutathione (GSH) trapped reactive metabolites from microsomal incubations are detected by this approach with a linear ion trap mass spectrometer [85]. Lim et al. also applied this approach for simultaneous detection and structural elucidation of GSH conjugates generated from human liver microsomal incubations by using LTQ/Orbitrap in a single run [86]. This approach is compound dependent and not suitable for various metabolites.

3.1.4 Pseudo neutral loss-dependent acquisition

This approach is based on neutral loss, which is a trigger for MS/MS acquisition. It is useful for the detection of metabolites, which shows neutral losses due to collision-induced dissociation. This approach consists of two full scans, one scan is at low collision energy (i.e., 5 eV) followed by a second scan with higher collision energy ramping (i.e., 20–40 eV), and spectra will be monitored for characteristic *m/z* differences of ion-pairs (neutral loss) between successive low and high collision energy full-scan MS. When such neutral losses are detected within a certain mass tolerance window, precursor ions will be identified from the low collision energy data and the instrument switches to MS/MS mode automatically to get the product ion spectra of those specific ions [87]. This approach is mainly useful for the phase II metabolites detection and characterization (e.g., neutral losses of 79.9568 for sulfate conjugates, 129.0426 for glutathione conjugates, and 176.0321 for glucuronide conjugates, etc.). The limitation of this approach is that it is unable to record MS/MS spectrum of metabolites with unpredictable fragmentation.

3.1.5 Mass defect-dependent acquisition

This approach is useful for the detection of both common and uncommon drug metabolites by using a mass defect filter (MDF). Interference ions from matrices are easily filtered out by MDF, because their mass defects are outside the mass defect range of common drug metabolites [88]. MDF is commonly used as a post-acquisition data processing technique and major instrument vendors are incorporating this in the metabolite identification software packages. In the TripleTOF® (Sciex) instrument, MDF is used as a selection factor to trigger MS/MS acquisition. Full-scan HRMS data are analyzed by applying real time MDF and identifies precursor ions whose mass defects fall within a specific window of a MDF. These ions are automatically followed by MS/MS acquisition. A different class of metabolites is detected by using multiple MDFs. Multiple mass defects are calculated by the software based on the elemental compositions of the parent, phase II conjugates, dealkylation, and hydrolysis metabolites and simultaneously perform the multiple mass filtering. This approach is useful for the rapid identification of drug metabolites in complex biological samples [89].

3.2 Data mining techniques for drug metabolite identification

Data interpretation is also an important step in drug metabolite identification and is a time-consuming process. Data mining techniques have been used to reduce the time required for data interpretation and to simplify the process of metabolite identification. Data mining involves software assisted post-acquisition data processing of the acquired data to obtain more accurate and rapid results. Different data mining techniques used for metabolite identification are extracted ion chromatogram, mass defect filter, product ion filter, neutral loss filter, isotope pattern filter, background subtraction, and control sample comparison [90].

3.2.1 Extracted ion chromatogram

In the extracted ion chromatogram (EIC) technique, expected metabolites are determined based on the predicted molecular masses of the metabolites. This technique first involves the acquisition of full scan in LC–MS/MS instrument and then application of ion extraction window to the acquired full-scan MS data-sets for identification of desired metabolite ion chromatogram [71]. Application of the narrow ion extraction window to the acquired MS datasets improves the sensitivity and selectivity. A narrow ion extraction window also helps in reducing false positive signals by removing the interferences from the ions outside of ion extraction window [91]. The limitation of this technique is unsuitability for the detection of metabolites with an unpredictable molecular mass.

3.2.2 Mass defect filter

Mass defect filter (MDF) is a software-based data filter technique developed for the detection of metabolites using full-scan HR-MS data. In this approach, metabolite ions will be differentiated from matrix ions based on the mass defect value of metabolites from their parent drug. Mass defect is defined as the difference between the exact mass and nominal mass of an element (e.g., ^{1}H and ^{14}N have an exact mass of 1.0078 and 14.00307 Da and nominal mass of 1 and 14 Da, therefore the calculated mass defect of ^{1}H and ^{14}N is +7.8 and + 3.07 mDa, respectively). It is based on the understanding that mass defect values of metabolites fall within a defined narrow window related to that of the parent drug. A narrow mass defect window (40–50 mDa) of MDF removes unwanted signals and causes enrichment of metabolites [91].

Phase I and Phase II metabolites are generally having mass defect values of less than 50 mDa relative to that of the structure of the parent drug. MDF has been applied for the identification of drug metabolites in plasma, urine, feces, bile, and in incubates of liver microsomes and hepatocytes [62, 92, 93]. All the metabolites generated are not structurally similar to the parent drug, some varies slightly (e.g., oxidation), and some show a significant variation (e.g., GSH adduct 68 mDa). If the MDF window is set at ±50 mDa, it excludes all the metabolites which have a mass defect value of more than 50 mDa and if the MDF window is broader, interference ions from the endogenous matrix will be included. So as to avoid it, multiple narrow MDF windows are developed and applied over a certain mass range. Drug filter, substructure filter, and conjugate filter are the commonly used MDF templates. Structures of metabolites that are generated by oxidation or reduction are slightly different from their parent drug structure for such type of metabolites, drug filter template is used. Metabolites that are generated by cleavage of the drug molecule are substructure metabolites of the parent drug compound, for such types of metabolites substructure filters are used. Metabolites that are generated due to conjugation reactions (phase II biotransformation reactions) are called conjugation metabolites, for this type of metabolites conjugate filter templates are used.

3.2.3 Product ion filter (PIF) and NL filter (NLF)

The mechanism for the identification of metabolites by PIF and NLF is based on the predicted product ion and predicted neutral loss fragmentation, respectively. Both known and unknown metabolites are determined by using these techniques. High-resolution product ion filter (PIF) and high-resolution neutral loss filter (NLF) are highly selective and sensitive techniques, and sometimes these are helpful to determine the trace amounts of unexpected metabolites that are not detected by MDF [94].

PIF is like a precursor ion filter scanning, a data acquisition technique, but PIF is a post-acquisition data mining technique, and metabolites are identified by applying multiple filters. On the other hand, multiple injections are required for the detection of multiple metabolites by precursor ion filter scanning. Likewise, NLF is like a neutral loss scanning; but the difference is avoiding the use of multiple injections because multiple filters are used to identify multiple desired metabolites [94, 95]. PIF and NLF are commonly used for the identification of Phase II metabolites (conjugated metabolites) [85, 96, 97].

3.2.4 Isotope pattern filtering (IPF)

This technique is useful for the identification of unexpected metabolites which have a distinct isotopic pattern. Metabolite ions that have a distinct isotopic pattern are extracted by applying the filters to full MS scan data. Most of the background peaks are eliminated by isotope pattern filtering (IPF) because many of the endogenous components do not show isotopic patterns [71]. IPF is applicable to the compounds containing distinct natural isotopes (Cl or Br) or synthetically incorporated isotopes (^{2}H,^{13}C and ^{15}N), or radiolabeled compound (^{14}C) with a distinct isotopic pattern. IPF is a valuable data mining tool for the identification and characterization of conjugated metabolites and reactive metabolites with improved selectivity and sensitivity [98–100].

3.2.5 Background subtraction

Background subtraction is an untargeted data mining technique in which the control and sample datasets are compared, and meticulously subtracted the background noise signals and matrix-related ion signals from the sample datasets. This technique finds the ions that are present in the test sample but not in a control sample. Control sample background subtraction algorithm is developed by Zhang *et al.* for complete removal of the matrix-related signals from the LC–MS/MS analyte dataset and isolation of the metabolite ions of interest. This algorithm is successfully applied for the identification of glutathione (GSH)-reactive metabolites [101].

Background signals from biological matrices and electrical noises were not efficiently removed by the background subtraction alone. To improve the efficiency, Zhu *et al.* developed a retention-time-shift-tolerant background subtraction and noise reduction algorithm (BgS-NoRA) for biological matrices [102]. The addition of noise reduction algorithm to background subtraction algorithm helps in the reduction of unwanted background signals (matrix-related ions) as well as electrical noises in biological matrices.

The limitation of this technique is a requirement of a good control sample containing all the possible matrix signals, and the consistency of run to run chromatographic retention time [101, 103, 104].

3.2.6 Control sample comparison

Control sample comparison is also an untargeted data mining technique in which control is compared with the sample. Metabolite ion chromatographic peaks are checked for their absence in the control sample. This process is tedious and challenging as the drug related metabolites are identified by comparing each metabolite ion in the spectrum of the analyte sample to that of the control sample. This technique is suitable for the identification of all types of metabolites but compared with the background subtraction, this is a less sensitive and selective technique [71, 91, 105].

4. Conclusions

In vitro metabolic stability studies are very important during drug discovery and development to predict the *in vivo* clearance of compounds and to know the number and types of metabolites formed. These studies are also helpful to find out the pharmacological and toxicological profiles of new chemical entities. *In vitro* metabolic stability studies are commonly performed by using liver microsomes and hepatocytes. LC-HRMS has turn into an important tool for the detection and characterization of drug metabolites *in vitro* and in complex biological samples. LC-HRMS, along with data acquisition and post-acquisition data mining techniques facilitated the drug metabolite identification.

Author details

Marothu Vamsi Krishna*, Kantamaneni Padmalatha and Gorrepati Madhavi
Vijaya Institute of Pharmaceutical Sciences for Women, Vijayawada, AP, India

*Address all correspondence to: vkmarothu@gmail.com

References

[1] Sheweita SA. Drug-metabolizing enzymes: mechanisms and functions. Current drug metabolism. 2000; 1(2):107-132.

[2] Baranczewski P, Stanczak A, Sundberg K, Svensson R, WallinA, Jansson J, Garberg P, Postlind H. Introduction to *in vitro* estimation of metabolic stability and drug interactions of new chemical entities in drug discovery and development. Pharmacological reports. 2006;58(4):453.

[3] Laine R. Metabolic stability: main enzymes involved and best tools to assess it. Current drug metabolism. 2008;9(9):921-927.

[4] Martiny VY, Miteva MA. Advances in molecular modeling of human cytochrome P450 polymorphism. Journal of molecular biology. 2013;425(21):3978-3992.

[5] Zanger UM, Schwab M. Cytochrome P450 enzymes in drug metabolism: regulation of gene expression, enzyme activities, and impact of genetic variation. Pharmacology & therapeutics. 2013;138(1):103-141.

[6] Kola I, Landis J. Can the pharmaceutical industry reduce attrition rates?. Nature reviews Drug discovery. 2004;3(8):711-716.

[7] Pelkonen O, Turpeinen M, Uusitalo J, Rautio A, Raunio H. Prediction of drug metabolism and interactions on the basis of *in vitro* investigations. Basic & clinical pharmacology & toxicology. 2005;96(3):167-175.

[8] Korfmacher WA. Advances in the integration of drug metabolism into the lead optimization paradigm. Mini reviews in medicinal chemistry. 2009;9(6):703-716.

[9] Li AP. Preclinical *in vitro* screening assays for drug-like properties. Drug discovery today: Technologies. 2005;2(2):179-185.

[10] Riley RJ, Grime K. Metabolic screening *in vitro*: metabolic stability, CYP inhibition and induction. Drug discovery today: Technologies.2004; 1(4):365-372.

[11] Barter ZE, Bayliss MK, Beaune PH, Boobis AR, Carlile DJ, Edwards RJ, Brian Houston J, Lake BG, Lipscomb JC, Pelkonen OR, Tucke GT. Scaling factors for the extrapolation of *in-vivo* metabolic drug clearance from *in vitro* data: reaching a consensus on values of human micro-somal protein and hepatocellularity per gram of liver. Current drug metabolism. 2007;8(1): 33-45.

[12] McNaney CA, Drexler DM, Hnatyshyn SY, Zvyaga TA, Knipe JO, Belcastro JV, Sanders M. An automated liquid chromatography-mass spectrometry process to determine metabolic stability half-life and intrinsic clearance of drug candidates by substrate depletion. Assay and drug development technologies. 2008;6(1):121-129.

[13] Chao P, Uss AS, Cheng KC. Use of intrinsic clearance for prediction of human hepatic clearance. Expert opinion on drug metabolism & toxicology. 2010;6(2):189-198.

[14] Słoczyńska K, Gunia-Krzyżak A, Koczurkiewicz P, Wójcik-Pszczoła K, Żelaszczyk D, Popiół J, Pękala E. Metabolic stability and its role in the discovery of new chemical entities. Actapharmaceutica. 2019;69(3): 345-361.

[15] Singh JK, Solanki A, Shirsath VS. Comparative *in vitro* intrinsic clearance of imipramine in multiple species liver

microsomes: human, rat, mouse and dog. Drug metabolism & toxicology. 2012;3(4).

[16] Basavapathruni A, Olhava EJ, Daigle SR, Therkelsen CA, Jin L, Boriack-Sjodin PA, Allain CJ, Klaus CR, Raimondi A, Scott MP, Dovletoglou A. Nonclinical pharmacokinetics and metabolism of EPZ-5676, a novel DOT1L histone methyltransferase inhibitor. Biopharmaceutics & drug disposition. 2014;35(4):237-252.

[17] Obach RS, Baxter JG, Liston TE, Silber BM, Jones BC, Macintyre F, Rance DJ, Wastall P. The prediction of human pharmacokinetic parameters from preclinical and *in vitro* metabolism data. Journal of pharmacology and experimental therapeutics. 1997;283(1):46-58.

[18] Lin JH, Chiba M, Balani SK, Chen IW, Kwei GY, Vastag KJ, Nishime JA. Species differences in the pharmacokinetics and metabolism of indinavir, a potent human immunodeficiency virus protease inhibitor. Drug metabolism and disposition. 1996;24(10):1111-1120.

[19] Obach RS. The importance of nonspecific binding in *in vitro* matrices, its impact on enzyme kinetic studies of drug metabolism reactions, and implications for *in vitro-in vivo* correlations. Drug metabolism and disposition. 1996;24:1047-1049.

[20] Liu F, Zhuang X, Yang C, Li Z, Xiong S, Zhang Z, Li J, Lu C, Zhang Z. Characterization of preclinical*in vitro* and *in vivo* ADME properties and prediction of human PK using a physiologically based pharmacokinetic model for YQA-14, a new dopamine D3 receptor antagonist candidate for treatment of drug addiction. Biopharmaceutics & drug disposition. 2014;35(5):296-307.

[21] Huang Z, Li H, Zhang Q, Tan X, Lu F, Liu H, Li S. Characterization of preclinical *in vitro* and *in vivo* pharmacokinetics properties for KBP-7018, a new tyrosine kinase inhibitor candidate for treatment of idiopathic pulmonary fibrosis. Drug design, development and therapy. 2015;9:4319-4328.

[22] Shah P, Kerns E, Nguyen DT, Obach RS, Wang AQ, Zakharov A, McKew J, Simeonov A, Hop CE, Xu X. An automated high-throughput metabolic stability assay using an integrated high-resolution accurate mass method and automated data analysis software. Drug metabolism and disposition. 2016;44(10):1653-1661.

[23] Nassar AE, Kamel AM, Clarimont C. Improving the decision-making process in the structural modification of drug candidates: enhancing metabolic stability. Drug discovery today. 2004;9(23):1020-1028.

[24] Di L, Obach RS. Addressing the challenges of low clearance in drug research. The AAPS journal. 2015;17(2):352-357.

[25] Brandon EF, Raap CD, Meijerman I, Beijnen JH, Schellens JH. An update on *in vitro* test methods in human hepatic drug biotransformation research: pros and cons. Toxicology and applied pharmacology. 2003;189(3):233-246.

[26] Fagerholm U. Prediction of human pharmacokinetics—evaluation of methods for prediction of hepatic metabolic clearance. Journal of pharmacy and pharmacology. 2007;59(6):803-828.

[27] Richmond W, Wogan M, Isbell J, Gordon WP. Interstrain differences of in vitro metabolic stability and impact on early drug discovery. Journal of pharmaceutical sciences. 2010;99(11):4463-4468.

[28] Chan TS, Yu H, Moore A, Khetani SR, Tweedie D. Meeting the

challenge of predicting hepatic clearance of compounds slowly metabolized by cytochrome P450 using a novel hepatocyte model, HepatoPac. Drug metabolism and disposition. 2013;41(12):2024-2032.

[29] Kumar GN, Surapaneni S. Role of drug metabolism in drug discovery and development. Medicinal research reviews. 2001;21(5):397-411.

[30] Masimirembwa CM, Thompson R, Andersson TB. *In vitro* high throughput screening of compounds for favorable metabolic properties in drug discovery. Combinatorial chemistry & high throughput screening. 2001;4(3):245-263.

[31] Zhang H, Zhang D, Li W, Yao M, D'Arienzo C, Li YX, Ewing WR, Gu Z, Zhu Y, Murugesan N, Shyu WC. Reduction of site-specific CYP3A-mediated metabolism for dual angiotensin and endothelin receptor antagonists in various *in vitro* systems and in cynomolgus monkeys. Drug metabolism and disposition. 2007;35(5):795-805.

[32] Masimirembwa CM, Bredberg U, Andersson TB. Metabolic stability for drug discovery and development. Clinical pharmacokinetics. 2003;42(6):515-528.

[33] Thompson TN. Optimization of metabolic stability as a goal of modern drug design. Medicinal research reviews. 2001;21(5):412-449.

[34] Crommentuyn KM, Schellens JH, Van Den Berg JD, Beijnen JH. *In vitro* metabolism of anti-cancer drugs, methods and applications: paclitaxel, docetaxel, tamoxifen and ifosfamide. Cancer treatment reviews. 1998;24(5):345-366.

[35] Donato MT, Castell JV. Strategies and molecular probes to investigate the role of cytochrome P450 in drug metabolism. Clinical pharmacokinetics. 2003;42(2):153-178.

[36] Plant N. Strategies for using *in vitro* screens in drug metabolism. Drug discovery today. 2004;9(7):328-336.

[37] Pelkonen O, Tolonen A, Rousu T, Tursas L, Turpeinen M, Hokkanen J, Uusitalo J, d'Yvoire MB, Coecke S. Comparison of metabolic stability and metabolite identification of 55 ECVAM/ ICCVAM validation compounds between human and rat liver homogenates and microsomes-a preliminary analysis. ALTEX-Alternatives to animal experimentation. 2009;26(3):214-222.

[38] Wang L, Chiang C, Liang H, Wu H, Feng W, Quinney SK, Li J, Li L. How to choose *in vitro* systems to predict *in vivo* drug clearance: A system pharmacology perspective. BioMed research international. 2015. https://doi.org/10.1155/2015/857327.

[39] Jia L, Liu X. The conduct of drug metabolism studies considered good practice (II): *in vitro* experiments. Current drug metabolism. 2007;8(8):822-829.

[40] Poulin P, Kenny JR, Hop CE, Haddad S. *In vitro–in vivo* extrapolation of clearance: Modeling hepatic metabolic clearance of highly bound drugs and comparative assessment with existing calculation methods. Journal of pharmaceutical sciences. 2012;101(2):838-851.

[41] Ma S, K Chowdhury S, B Alton K. Application of mass spectrometry for metabolite identification. Current drug metabolism. 2006;7(5):503-523.

[42] Krueger P, Daneshfar R, Eckert GP, Klein J, Volmer DA, Bahr U, Müller WE, Karas M, Schubert-Zsilavecz M, Abdel-Tawab M. Metabolism of boswellic acids *in vitro* and *in vivo*. Drug metabolism and disposition. 2008;36(6):1135-1142.

[43] Mukkavilli R, Pinjari J, Patel B, Sengottuvelan S, Mondal S, Gadekar A, Verma M, Patel J, Pothuri L, Chandrashekar G, Koiram P. *In vitro* metabolism, disposition, preclinical pharmacokinetics and prediction of human pharmacokinetics of DNDI-VL-2098, a potential oral treatment for Visceral Leishmaniasis. European journal of pharmaceutical sciences. 2014;65:147-155.

[44] Ellefsen KN, Wohlfarth A, Swortwood MJ, Diao X, Concheiro M, Huestis MA. 4-Methoxy-α-PVP: in silico prediction, metabolic stability, and metabolite identification by human hepatocyte incubation and high-resolution mass spectrometry. Forensic toxicology. 2016;34(1):61-75.

[45] Pelkonen O, Kaltiala EH, Larmi TK, Kärki NT. Cytochrome P-450-linked monooxygenase system and drug-induced spectral interactions in human liver microsomes. Chemico-biological interactions. 1974;9(3):205-216.

[46] Eichelbaum M, Burk O. CYP3A genetics in drug metabolism. Nature medicine. 2001;7(3):285-287.

[47] Quintieri L, Fantin M, Palatini P, De Martin S, Rosato A, Caruso M, Geroni C, Floreani M. *In vitro* hepatic conversion of the anticancer agent nemorubicin to its active metabolite PNU-159682 in mice, rats and dogs: a comparison with human liver microsomes. Biochemical pharmacology. 2008;76(6):784-795.

[48] Li CM, Lu Y, Narayanan R, Miller DD, Dalton JT. Drug metabolism and pharmacokinetics of 4-substituted methoxybenzoyl-aryl-thiazoles. Drug metabolism and disposition. 2010;38(11):2032-2039.

[49] Di L, Kerns EH, Hong Y, Kleintop TA, Mc Connell OJ, Huryn DM. Optimization of a higher throughput microsomal stability screening assay for profiling drug discovery candidates. Journal of biomolecular screening. 2003;8(4):453-462.

[50] Huang J, Si L, Fan Z, Hu L, Qiu J, Li G. *In vitro* metabolic stability and metabolite profiling of TJ0711 hydrochloride, a newly developed vasodilatory β-blocker, using a liquid chromatography–tandem mass spectrometry method. Journal of chromatography B. 2011;879(30):3386-3392.

[51] Słoczyńska K, Pańczyk K, Waszkielewicz AM, Marona H, Pękala E. *In vitro* mutagenic, antimutagenic, and antioxidant activities evaluation and biotransformation of some bioactive 4-substituted 1-(2-methoxyphenyl) piperazine derivatives. Journal of biochemical and molecular toxicology. 2016;30(12):593-601.

[52] Waszkielewicz AM, Słoczyńska K, Pękala E, Żmudzki P, Siwek A, Gryboś A, Marona H. Design, synthesis, and anticonvulsant activity of some derivatives of xanthone with aminoalkanol moieties. Chemical biology & drug design. 2017;89(3):339-352.

[53] Knights KM, Stresser DM, Miners JO, Crespi CL. *In vitro* drug metabolism using liver microsomes. Current protocols in pharmacology. 2016;74(1):7.8.1-7.8.24.

[54] Gomez-Lechon MJ, Donato MT, Castell JV, Jover R. Human hepatocytes in primary culture: the choice to investigate drug metabolism in man. Current drug metabolism. 2004;5(5):443-462.

[55] Chenery RJ, Ayrton A, Oldham HG, Standring P, Norman SJ, Seddon T, Kirby R. Diazepam metabolism in cultured hepatocytes from rat, rabbit, dog, guinea pig, and man. Drug

metabolism and disposition. 1987; 15(3):312-317.

[56] Le Bigot JF, Begue JM, Kiechel JR, Guillouzo A. Species differences in metabolism of ketotifen in rat, rabbit and man: demonstration of similar pathways *in vivo* and in cultured hepatocytes. Life sciences. 1987;40(9):883-890.

[57] Berry MN, Halls HJ, Grivell MB. Techniques for pharmacological and toxicological studies with isolated hepatocyte suspensions. Life sciences. 1992;51(1):1-6.

[58] Cross DM, Bell JA, Wilson K. Kinetics of ranitidine metabolism in dog and rat isolated hepatocytes. Xenobiotica. 1995;25(4):367-375.

[59] Bayliss MK. Utility of hepatocytes to model species differences in the metabolism of loxtidine and to predict pharmacokinetic parameters in rat, dog and man. Xenobiotica. 1999;29(3):253-268.

[60] Lu C, Li P, Gallegos R, Uttamsingh V, Xia CQ, Miwa GT, Balani SK, Gan LS. Comparison of intrinsic clearance in liver microsomes and hepatocytes from rats and humans: evaluation of free fraction and uptake in hepatocytes. Drug metabolism and disposition. 2006;34(9):1600-1605.

[61] Zanelli U, Caradonna NP, Hallifax D, Turlizzi E, Houston JB. Comparison of cryopreserved HepaRG cells with cryopreserved human hepatocytes for prediction of clearance for 26 drugs. Drug metabolism and disposition. 2012;40(1):104-110.

[62] Gandhi AS, Wohlfarth A, Zhu M, Pang S, Castaneto M, Scheidweiler KB, Huestis MA. High-resolution mass spectrometric metabolite profiling of a novel synthetic designer drug, N-(adamantan-1-yl)-1-(5-fluoropentyl)-1H-indole-3-carboxamide (STS-135), using cryopreserved human hepatocytes and assessment of metabolic stability with human liver microsomes. Drug testing and analysis. 2015;7(3):187-198.

[63] McGinnity DF, Soars MG, Urbanowicz RA, Riley RJ. Evaluation of fresh and cryopreserved hepatocytes as *in vitro* drug metabolism tools for the prediction of metabolic clearance. Drug metabolism and disposition. 2004;32(11):1247-1253.

[64] Bungay PJ, Tweedy S, Howe DC, Gibson KR, Jones HM, Mount NM. Preclinical and clinical pharmacokinetics of PF-02413873, a nonsteroidal progesterone receptor antagonist. Drug metabolism and disposition. 2011;39(8):1396-1405.

[65] Klieber S, Arabeyre-Fabre C, Moliner P, Marti E, Mandray M, Ngo R, Ollier C, Brun P, Fabre G. Identification of metabolic pathways and enzyme systems involved in the *in vitro* human hepatic metabolism of dronedarone, a potent new oral antiarrhythmic drug. Pharmacology research & perspectives. 2014;2(3):e00044.

[66] Gómez-Lechón MJ, Castell JV, Donato MT. Hepatocytes—the choice to investigate drug metabolism and toxicity in man: *in vitro* variability as a reflection of *in vivo*. Chemico-biological interactions. 2007;168(1):30-50.

[67] Green MD, Yang X, Cramer M, King CD. *In vitro* metabolic studies on the selective metabotropic glutamate receptor sub-type 5 (mGluR5) antagonist 3-[(2-methyl-1, 3-thiazol-4-yl) ethynyl]-pyridine (MTEP). Neuroscience letters. 2006; 391(3):91-95.

[68] Rudraraju AV, Hossain MF, Shrestha A, Amoyaw PN, Tekwani BL. *In vitro* Metabolic Stability Study of New Cyclen Based Antimalarial Drug Leads Using RP-HPLC and LC-MS/MS.

Modern chemistryand applications. 2014;2(129):2.

[69] Asha S, Vidyavathi M. Role of human liver microsomes in *in vitro* metabolism of drugs—a review. Applied biochemistry and biotechnology. 2010;160(6):1699-1722.

[70] Sowjanya G, Ganapaty S, Sharma R. *In vitro* test methods for metabolite identification: A review. Asian journal of pharmacy and pharmacology. 2019;5(3):441-450.

[71] Zhu M, Zhang H, Humphreys WG. Drug metabolite profiling and identification by high-resolution mass spectrometry. Journal of biological chemistry. 2011;286(29):25419-25425.

[72] Tiller PR, Romanyshyn LA. Liquid chromatography/tandem mass spectrometric quantification with metabolite screening as a strategy to enhance the early drug discovery process. Rapid communications in mass spectrometry. 2002;16(12):1225-1231.

[73] Castro-Perez J, Plumb R, Granger JH, Beattie I, Joncour K, Wright A. Increasing throughput and information content for *in vitro* drug metabolism experiments using ultra-performance liquid chromatography coupled to a quadrupole time-of-flight mass spectrometer. Rapid communications in mass spectrometry. 2005;19(6):843-848.

[74] Blair IA. Applications of mass spectrometry to toxicology. Chemical research in toxicology. 1993;6(6):741-747.

[75] Baillie TA, Davis MR. Mass spectrometry in the analysis of glutathione conjugates. Biological mass spectrometry. 1993;22(6):319-325.

[76] Ma S, Chowdhury SK. Application of liquid chromatography/mass spectrometry for metabolite identification. In: Drug Metabolism in Drug Design and Development: Basic Concepts and Practice (Zhang D, Zhu M, Humphreys WG, editors.) John Wiley & Sons, 2007, pp. 319-367.

[77] Ma S, Chowdhury SK. Data acquisition and data mining techniques for metabolite identification using LC coupled to high-resolution MS. Bioanalysis. 2013;5(10):1285-1297.

[78] Xie C, Zhong D, Yu K, Chen X. Recent advances in metabolite identification and quantitative bioanalysis by LC–Q-TOF MS. Bioanalysis. 2012;4(8):937-959.

[79] Andrews GL, Simons BL, Young JB, Hawkridge AM, Muddiman DC. Performance characteristics of a new hybrid quadrupole time-of-flight tandem mass spectrometer (TripleTOF 5600). Analytical chemistry. 2011;83(13):5442-5446.

[80] Perry RH, Cooks RG, Noll RJ. Orbitrap mass spectrometry: instrumentation, ion motion and applications. Mass spectrometry reviews. 2008;27(6):661-699.

[81] Makarov A, Denisov E, Kholomeev A, Balschun W, Lange O, Strupat K, Horning S. Performance evaluation of a hybrid linear ion trap/orbitrap mass spectrometer. Analytical chemistry. 2006;78(7):2113-2120.

[82] Peterman SM, Duczak N, Kalgutkar AS, Lame ME, Soglia JR. Application of a linear ion trap/orbitrap mass spectrometer in metabolite characterization studies: examination of the human liver microsomal metabolism of the non-tricyclic anti-depressant nefazodone using data-dependent accurate mass measurements. Journal of the American society for mass spectrometry. 2006;17(3):363-375.

[83] Anari MR, Sanchez RI, Bakhtiar R, Franklin RB, Baillie TA. Integration of

knowledge-based metabolic predictions with liquid chromatography data-dependent tandem mass spectrometry for drug metabolism studies: application to studies on the biotransformation of indinavir. Analytical chemistry. 2004;76(3):823-832.

[84] Lim HK, Chen J, Sensenhauser C, Cook K, Subrahmanyam V. Metabolite identification by data-dependent accurate mass spectrometric analysis at resolving power of 60 000 in external calibration mode using an LTQ/Orbitrap. Rapid communications in mass spectrometry, 2007; 21(12):1821-1832.

[85] Ma L, Wen B, Ruan Q, Zhu M. Rapid screening of glutathione-trapped reactive metabolites by linear ion trap mass spectrometry with isotope pattern-dependent scanning and post-acquisition data mining. Chemical research in toxicology. 2008; 21(7):1477-1483.

[86] Lim HK, Chen J, Cook K, Sensenhauser C, Silva J, Evans DC. A generic method to detect electrophilic intermediates using isotopic pattern triggered data-dependent high-resolution accurate mass spectrometry. Rapid communications in mass spectrometry, 2008;22(8):1295-1311.

[87] Castro-Perez J, Plumb R, Liang L, Yang E. A high-throughput liquid chromatography/tandem mass spectrometry method for screening glutathione conjugates using exact mass neutral loss acquisition. Rapid communications in mass spectrometry, 2005;19(6):798-804.

[88] Zhu M, Ma L, Zhang D, Ray K, Zhao W, Humphreys WG, Skiles G, Sanders M, Zhang H. Detection and characterization of metabolites in biological matrices using mass defect filtering of liquid chromatography/high resolution mass spectrometry data. Drug metabolism and disposition. 2006;34(10):1722-1733.

[89] Campbell JL, Le Blanc JY. Using high-resolution quadrupole TOF technology in DMPK analyses. Bioanalysis. 2012;4(5):487-500.

[90] Dhurjad PS, Marothu VK, Rathod R. Post-acquisition data mining techniques for LC–MS/MS-acquired data in drug metabolite identification. Bioanalysis. 2017;9(16):1265-1278.

[91] Wen B, Zhu M. Applications of mass spectrometry in drug metabolism: 50 years of progress. Drug metabolism reviews. 2015;47(1):71-87.

[92] Yang A, Zang M, Liu H, Fan P, Xing J. Metabolite identification of the antimalarial piperaquine*in vivo* using liquid chromatography–high-resolution mass spectrometry in combination with multiple data-mining tools in tandem. Biomedical chromatography. 2016;30(8):1324-1330.

[93] Kalariya PD, Patel PN, Kavya P, Sharma M, Garg P, Srinivas R, Talluri MK. Rapid structural characterization of *in vivo* and *in vitro* metabolites of tinoridine using UHPLC–QTOF–MS/MS and in silico toxicological screening of its metabolites. Journal of mass spectrometry. 2015;50(11):1222-1233.

[94] Ruan Q, Peterman S, Szewc MA, Ma L, Cui D, Humphreys WG, Zhu M. An integrated method for metabolite detection and identification using a linear ion trap/Orbitrap mass spectrometer and multiple data processing techniques: application to indinavir metabolite detection. Journal of mass spectrometry. 2008;43(2):251-261.

[95] Zhang H, Zhu M. Drug metabolite identification with high-resolution mass spectrometry. In: Handbook of Metabolic Pathways of Xenobiotics (1st edition). Lee PW (Ed.). John Wiley & Sons, NJ, USA, 2014, 1-23.

[96] Wrona M, Mauriala T, Bateman KP, Mortishire-Smith RJ, O'Connor D. All-in-one'analysis for metabolite identification using liquid chromatography/hybrid quadrupole time-of-flight mass spectrometry with collision energy switching. Rapid communications in mass spectrometry, 2005;19(18):2597-2602.

[97] Yao M, Ma L, Duchoslav E, Zhu M. Rapid screening and characterization of drug metabolites using multiple ion monitoring dependent product ion scan and post-acquisition data mining on a hybrid triple quadrupole-linear ion trap mass spectrometer. Rapid communications in mass spectrometry. 2009;23(11):1683-1693.

[98] Zhu P, Tong W, Alton K, Chowdhury S. An accurate-mass-based spectral-averaging isotope-pattern-filtering algorithm for extraction of drug metabolites possessing a distinct isotope pattern from LC-MS data. Analytical chemistry. 2009;81(14): 5910-5917.

[99] LeBlanc A, Shiao TC, Roy R, Sleno L. Improved detection of reactive metabolites with a bromine-containing glutathione analog using mass defect and isotope pattern matching. Rapid communications in mass spectrometry, 2010;24(9):1241-1250.

[100] Du F, Ruan Q, Zhu M, Xing J. Detection and characterization of ticlopidine conjugates in rat bile using high-resolution mass spectrometry: applications of various data acquisition and processing tools. Journal of mass spectrometry. 2013;48(3):413-422.

[101] Zhang H, Yang Y. An algorithm for thorough background subtraction from high-resolution LC/MS data: application for detection of glutathione-trapped reactive metabolites. Journal of mass spectrometry. 2008;43(9):1181-1190.

[102] Zhu P, Ding W, Tong W, Ghosal A, Alton K, Chowdhury S. Aretention-time-shift-tolerant background subtraction and noise reduction algorithm (BgS-NoRA) for extraction of drug metabolites in liquid chromatography/mass spectrometry data from biological matrices. Rapid communications in mass spectrometry. 2009;23(11):1563-1572.

[103] Jhajra S, Prasad B, Shah J, Singh S. High-resolution MS for drug metabolite identification. In: Applications of High-Resolution Mass Spectrometry in Drug Discovery and Development. Sleno L (Ed.). Future Science Group, London, UK, 2013, 22-40.

[104] Xing J, Zang M, Zhang H, Zhu M. The application of high-resolution mass spectrometry-based data-mining tools in tandem to metabolite profiling of a triple drug combination in humans. Analyticachimicaacta. 2015;897:34-44.

[105] Barbara JE, Castro-Perez JM. High-resolution chromatography/time-of-flight MSE with in silico data mining is an information-rich approach to reactive metabolite screening. Rapid communications in mass spectrometry. 2011;25(20):3029-3040.